# Health *Scents*

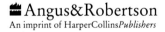

A L A N   H A Y E S

**Angus&Robertson**
An imprint of HarperCollins*Publishers*

**Note:** *Neither the author nor the publisher directly or indirectly dispense medical advice or prescribe the use of various herbal remedies. The intent is to provide information that you may wish to explore as a natural alternative. Information about the use of some essential oils can be found on pages 40–43. Information about when to avoid massage can be found on page 64. If you have any queries, you should seek the advice of your medical practitioner.*

***Angus&Robertson***
*An imprint of HarperCollins Publishers, Australia*

*First published in Australia in 1995*

**HarperCollins Publishers**
*25–31 Ryde Road, Pymble, NSW 2073, Australia*
*31 View Road, Glenfield, Auckland 10, New Zealand*
*77–85 Fulham Palace Road, London W6 8JB, United Kingdom*
*Hazelton Lanes, 55 Avenue Road, Suite 2900, Toronto, Ontario M5R 3L2*
*and 1995 Markham Road, Scarborough, Ontario M1B 5M8, Canada*
*10 East 53rd Street, New York NY 10022, USA*

*National Library of Australia Cataloguing-in-Publication data:*

*Hayes, Alan B. (Alan Bruce), 1949-*
*Health scents*

*ISBN 0 207 18229 9*
*1. Aromatherapy. I. Title.*
*615.321*

*Printed in Hong Kong*

*5 4 3 2 1   95 96 97 98*

# *Contents*

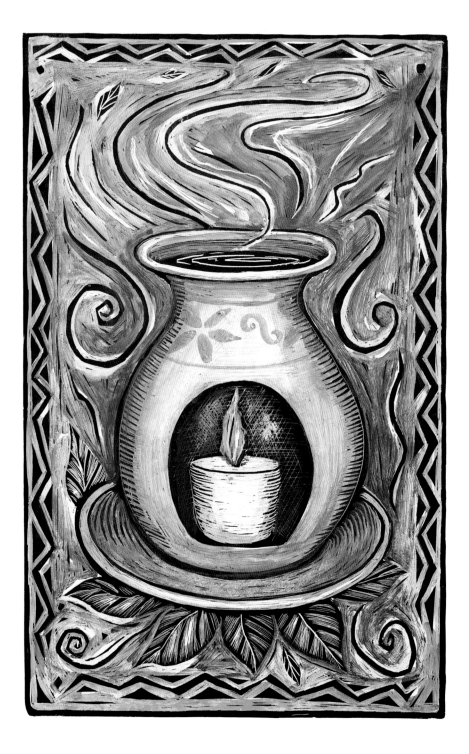

# Introduction

Aromatherapy is the art of using fragrant essential oils, derived from the odoriferous part of plants, to restore vitality to the body and to enhance health and appearance.

The ancient Chinese are generally acknowledged as being the first civilisation in recorded history to practice aromatherapy. However, it is likely that the benefits of essential oils were known long before this. Indeed, the use of aromatic substances certainly flourished during the time of the ancient Egyptians. Translations of hieroglyphics found in ancient tombs and temples reveal that extracted aromatics were used in various medicinal preparations to treat a variety of illnesses.

Greek physicians visiting Egypt acquired the knowledge of using essential oils, and discovered that highly aromatic plants possessed stimulating or edifying properties. The Arabs first extracted essential oils from plants around the 10th century and used them for medicinal purposes. The Knights of the Crusades brought these aromatic essences back to Europe, having successfully used the healing properties of certain plant oils, such as oil of St John's wort, to treat their battle wounds.

The burning of essential oils in fragrant candles and aromatic woods became commonplace during the bubonic plague of 14th century England to combat infection and to mask the stench of death. Even today hospitals and homes burn aromatic oils because of their antibacterial properties.

By the end of the 18th century, essential oils were being used widely in medicinal preparations. They continued to be used extensively until it was discovered that synthetic laboratory substitutes could be produced more quickly and cheaply. These synthetic versions are still used to this day in many of our perfumes and medicines. However, while they may smell like the real thing, they do not possess those important therapeutic properties.

Today pure essential oils are once again being used for health and healing. Their popularity may be attributed to the efforts of Dr Jean Valnet, a French doctor who used them to treat soldier's wounds and infections during World War II. He firmly believed that natural essences were far superior to any synthetic version, a view shared by his close colleague, biochemist Marguerite Maury. She was convinced that essential oils could be beneficial in skin care, in particular in delaying the ageing process and solving stress-related problems. It was Maury's work and techniques that created the foundations of modern aromatherapy.

To enjoy the many benefits of essentials oils, one does not need to be a practitioner or to embark upon an extensive course of training (although you may find that this book will initiate such a desire!). The only criterion is a passion for the aromatic pleasure and therapeutic value that can be gained from using essential oils.

This book will lead you through the many advantages of incorporating different aromatic oils in your daily life. They may be used to soothe the nerves, fight infection and aid the healing process, or just to arouse the senses, revitalise your body and soul and provide sheer hedonistic pleasure.

You will be shown how and why essential oils work, and how they are best used or applied. There are easy to follow instructions for blending your own perfumes and tips on choosing oils to create 'scentsational'

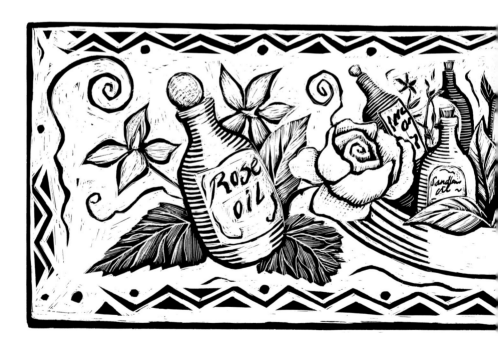

magic. You will enter the fragrant world of 'flower power', and learn why it affects your feelings and memory. And, for those who enjoy the magic of touch, there are recipes for sensual massage oils to 'set the mood', to restore the body and relieve stress and anxiety, and to ease the distress of pain.

The face, neck, lips, arms, legs and feet can all be nourished and pampered with essential oils, used either alone or in cleansers, tonics and moisturising creams or lotions. And, just for women, there are certain essential oils which are useful for treating problems which may occur during menstruation, menopause or pregnancy, such as sore breasts and nipples.

If you have a hot tub or jacuzzi, you will find that soothing essential oils are the perfect partner to the hot, swirling water at the end of a hectic day. And, to tease and tantalise the senses, this book also includes recipes for aromatic air freshener sprays, oils for burning, fragrant candles, perfumed pillows and bed linen and even a section on edible essential oils.

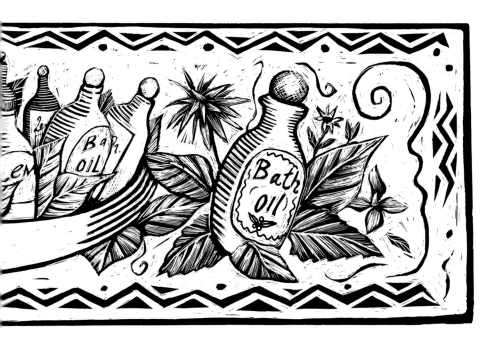

# CHAPTER ONE

# Medicines From the Earth

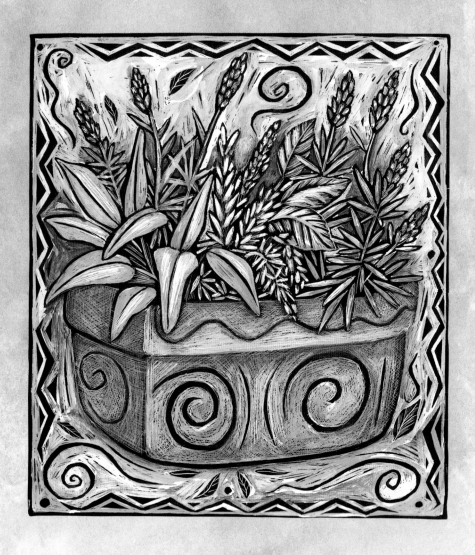

# Essential Oils, Their Properties and Uses

Essential oils are highly scented, volatile plant hormones which, when absorbed into the bloodstream, can renew and maintain good health. Whether you inhale them, add them to the bath, dab them on your skin, or include them in a massage oil, their beneficial properties can make you feel terrific.

The rich perfumes of essential oils can calm, soothe, heal, fight infection, revitalise, relax and stimulate the body. The oils are very concentrated so only a small amount, just a few drops, is usually necessary.

## Soothing the Nerves

Essential oils are valued for their ability to redress any imbalance between the two parts of the autonomic nervous system: that is, the sympathetic and the parasympathetic nerves.

## Fighting Infection

The antibacterial constituents of certain essential oils make them useful in both treating and preventing infection, by helping to boost the body's resistance. One of the strongest natural antiseptics is eucalyptus oil, which contains the potent and powerful antibacterial constituent, eucalyptol. Other potent antiseptic oils are lemon, pine, clove, thyme and cinnamon.

## Healing

Essential oils appear to work by speeding up the process of cellular regeneration, thus helping the skin to heal faster. Some oils — thyme, sage and rosemary in particular — have anti-inflammatory properties, making them useful not only for treating sores, cuts, burns and bruises, but in relieving the pain of arthritis and rheumatism. Lavender oil, for instance, can be used to relieve the pain of a headache. Simply massage a couple of drops of the oil into your temples with your fingertips.

Other oils can aid in the treatment of injuries, such as sprains, strains and torn ligaments. Essential oils such as hyssop, oregano and St John's wort can be used to relieve aches and pains and to relax stiff muscles.

## Skin and Hair Care

Several essential oils are particularly beneficial to the skin and may be used to treat hair and scalp conditions. They can be included in creams and lotions, aromatic baths and showers, shampoos and hair and scalp conditioning oils.

## Revitalisation

Research has shown that essential oils affect the body's hormone-producing glands and that, after entering the bloodstream, the organs absorb them as they do other nutrients. In this way specific oils can then regulate certain problems. For example, anise and mint stimulate the pituitary gland, which in turn affects most of the other hormone-producing glands. Lavender oil rubbed onto the wrists or the nape of the neck has a calming effect. Other oils such as cinnamon and ylang-ylang, have natural aphrodisiac properties and are reputed to revive a waning sex drive.

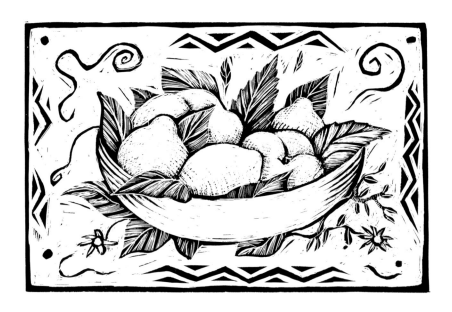

# *How Do Essential Oils Work?*

There are two ways in which essential oils work to heal and revitalise the body. One is by smell, and the other is by entering the whole body system and bloodstream (usually through the lungs by inhalation, and through the skin from massage, baths and compresses).

All of the essential oils have different fragrances — some are menthol-like, while others are flowery or zesty and refreshing. When we smell them they have an immediate effect on our autonomic nervous system and hormonal system. It is these systems that govern our reactions, such as fear or anger, our memory, stress levels and heart rate.

Our sense of smell has a powerful effect on our minds and bodies. Aromatherapy recognises this attribute and uses it accordingly. An example is the heady scent of jasmine, which can both soothe and uplift the senses, while the fragrance of basil will clear the head. So we can see how the scents of different essential oils can evoke different responses or states of mind, from calming and sedating our bodies after a tiring day to mental revival and restoration.

As the essential oils enter the body system, they are transported by the circulation of the blood to the various organs, which benefit from the oils' therapeutic effect. Some oils have an affinity with a particular organ and organs or glands in need of help will selectively take up the appropriate oil. It will then remain there for a number of hours and trigger off a healing process which can continue for a number of days. Any oil that cannot be utilised is eliminated via exhalation, perspiration, or the urine and faeces.

The benefits of aromatherapy oils are many and varied. It is a treatment that will relax both the mind and the body, resulting in improved skin and circulation, a stronger immune system and increased levels of vitality and overall wellbeing.

Essential oils can assist with acute and chronic illness, heighten the body's ability to cope with stress, act as a natural antiseptic to prevent infection, help to speed up the healing process, detoxify the body, exert antibiotic and antiviral properties, and soothe the nervous system.

# Application of Essential Oils

Oils can be used or applied in the following ways:

## Massage

This is the most common method of applying the essential oils used in the practice of aromatherapy. The oils enter the body and then the bloodstream through this contact with every part of the skin.

A good massage is an effective and drug-free therapy that enhances circulation and improves skin and muscle tone. It can relieve painful joints and muscles, help reduce tension and high blood pressure, stimulate the immune system and clear away fatigue-producing chemicals, leaving the nerve endings of the skin soothed and relaxed.

In the bedroom, aromatic and sensual massage can enhance your love life by improving both your disposition and general wellbeing. It will give pleasure to you and your partner, and make your lovemaking far more enjoyable, exciting and fulfilling.

## In the Bath

The bath is the perfect place to unwind and renew body energy. Essential oils added to your bath water release special properties which penetrate your skin, and also exert their therapeutic benefits through the vapour you inhale.

For maximum effect, close all windows and the bathroom door. If you are ill, nauseated or running a fever it is not advisable to take a full bath: instead, just sponge down underarms and genitals with a little of the scented water. However, a therapeutic bath can do wonders in speeding up recovery if you are suffering from a cold or stuffed up nose, aching muscles and joints, or just when you feel tired and run down.

Before you add any essential oils to your bath, consider first how you feel at present and then how you would like to feel. Then consult the section *A Guide to Essential Oils* (see page 37) and choose the appropriate blend.

To make a bath oil, dilute 10 drops of essential oil with 35 ml (1 fl oz) of almond oil and 5 ml (⅙ fl oz) of wheat germ oil. Store in an airtight, amber-coloured glass bottle. Add about 10 drops of the oil mix to the bath while the taps are running, either singly or in the following suggested combinations:

## TO REVITALISE AFTER A BUSY DAY

*5 drops bergamot essential oil*
*5 drops ylang-ylang essential oil*

This is the perfect combination after a busy day, particularly if you still have to go out that evening. Add to a warm bath and relax in it for 10 minutes.

## TO REVITALISE AND RESTORE HEALTH

*10 drops tangerine essential oil*

This oil is ideal for restoring energy levels, especially after illness.

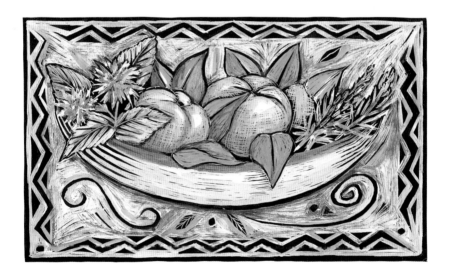

## TO CALM AND RELAX

*4 drops lime flower essential oil*
*2 drops rosemary essential oil*
*2 drops bay essential oil*
*2 drops pennyroyal essential oil*

Use this blend to calm down and relax after a hard day at school or work.

### A RELAXING EVENING BATH

*6 drops lavender essential oil*
*2 drops chamomile essential oil*
*2 drops rose essential oil*

### TO RELAX AND UNWIND

*5 drops lavender essential oil*
*5 drops rosewood essential oil*

### TO RELAX, SOOTHE AND PROMOTE SLEEP

*6 drops chamomile essential oil*
*2 drops lovage essential oil*
*2 drops lime flower essential oil*

### TO SOOTHE DEPRESSING MOODS

#### MELANCHOLY

*10 drops of either rose, neroli or chamomile essential oil*

#### ANXIETY

*10 drops of either chamomile, neroli o lavender essential oil*

#### ANGER

*10 drops of either rose or chamomile essential oil*

### A REFRESHING SUMMER BATH

*10 drops of either peppermint or lemon essential oil*

### TO EASE TIRED AND ACHING MUSCLES

*4 drops hyssop essential oil*
*2 drops rosemary essential oil*
*2 drops bay essential oil*
*2 drops rose essential oil*

### TO RELIEVE STIFFNESS FROM SPORT

*5 drops hyssop essential oil*
*5 drops rosemary essential oil*
*2 drops bay essential oil*

### AN INVIGORATING AND REJUVENATING BATH

*6 drops lavender essential oil*
*2 drops rosewood or lovage essential oil*
*2 drops tangerine essential oil*

### A SPECIAL BATH FOR COLDS

With this blend the essential oils need not be mixed with a carrier oil, but should be added straight to the bath water.

*6 drops pine essential oil*
*6 drops eucalyptus essential oil*
*6 drops cypress essential oil*

Run the water as hot as you can stand it and, when the bath is almost full, add the essential oils.

Sit with your knees up and your head between them so that you can fully inhale the restorative vapours. As the water cools, slosh it all over your body. Get out, dry yourself vigorously with a warm towel, and then wrap yourself in another warm towel for a few minutes.

To finish off, rub your entire body with this mixture of oils:

*80 ml (2½ fl oz) almond oil*
*35 ml (1 fl oz) hazelnut oil*
*5 ml (⅙ fl oz) wheat germ oil*
*3 drops lavender essential oil*
*2 drops eucalyptus essential oil*
*2 drops thyme essential oil*

## Aromatic Showers

Even if your daily schedule does not allow time for a relaxing bath, you can still enjoy the benefits of fragrant essential oils with an aromatic shower. To begin, rub your entire body with a little bath oil of your choice, diluted 50:50 with water. Plug the shower drain and, while showering, sprinkle in the same aromatics as the water collects.

### BODY MASSAGE OIL

Apply immediately after bath or shower after thoroughly towel drying.

*85 ml (3 fl oz) almond oil*
*40 ml (1½ fl oz) hazelnut oil*
*25 ml (1 fl oz) jojoba oil*
*5 ml (⅙ fl oz) essential oil of your choice*
*(select from* A Guide to Essential Oils *[page 37])*

Combine all ingredients in an amber-coloured glass bottle and seal tightly. Shake vigorously until the oils are well blended.

To apply a massage oil after the shower or bath, follow these tips:

❋ *Pour a teaspoon of the oil into your palm, rub your hands together, and then apply it to the breasts and buttocks with a circular motion.*

❋ *Using a small amount of additional oil, rub your solar plexus six times in an anticlockwise direction. Then stroke the remaining oil upwards over your stomach, using both hands.*

❋ *Pour another teaspoon of oil into your palm, rub your hands together, and massage each arm with long, firm strokes from the hand to the shoulder. Finish off by kneading deeply, yet gently, up your arm with your fingertips.*

✳ *Using one more teaspoon of oil, work up your legs with deep, firm strokes. Move from each ankle to the top of each thigh, working with both hands.*

## Footbaths

Your feet communicate with the rest of your body, which is why a foot massage, combined with a therapeutic footbath, will revive your entire system.

You can choose from any of the oils listed in *A Guide to Essential Oils* (see page 37) or use the blend recommended in Chapter 4 (see page 62) for foot massages.

To soak your feet, you will need a basin large enough to hold them when they are fully stretched out. Pour in sufficient water to cover your ankles and select an essential oil or oil blend which is appropriate to how you feel. Add 3 to 4 drops to the water, or more if you do not feel it is sufficiently scented.

Before soaking your feet, give each one a preliminary massage.

## Saunas and Jacuzzis

Those of you who are fortunate enough to own a sauna or a jacuzzi have no doubt found that it is a marvellous haven in which to unwind and restore the body functions.

The whirlpool jets of a jacuzzi will gently massage the muscles, easing away any soreness and tension. The addition of essential oils will enhance the jacuzzi's ability to calm and soothe frazzled nerves, and to restore tired and aching bodies.

Saunas are extremely useful for eliminating toxins from the body. The inclusion of essential oils in a sauna will help promote this eliminative process, removing waste products and debris through the skin. Simply include the aromatic oils of your choice in the water that you throw on the coals, or other heat source. Mix 2 drops of essential oil with every 600 ml (20 fl oz) of water.

Ideal oils for use in a sauna are eucalyptus, pine and tea tree. They are all excellent cleansers and detoxifiers, entering the body by inhalation and exiting through perspiration. It must be remembered, though, that saunas can leave you a little depleted unless you drink fluids, preferably water, at the same time. Limit your time in the sauna to avoid possible dehydration.

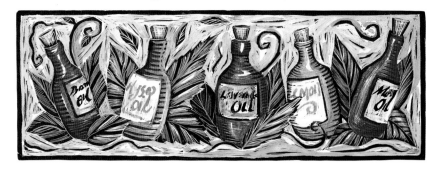

## A Word of Advice

Jacuzzis and saunas may both pose a health risk for people who suffer from heart or blood pressure problems. Those with heart problems could easily be affected by the sudden temperature changes from hot to cold, and back again. With each temperature change your heart rate can increase by at least 60% or more — as much as occurs with moderate exercise. Also, as you acclimatise to the higher temperatures, your blood pressure will drop. This is a definite risk to those over 50 years of age who are predisposed to arteriosclerosis, or who have a poorly functioning heart. Such a decline in blood pressure could be the catalyst for a mild stroke.

Consider the following before you make use of either jacuzzis or saunas:

❊ *What is your general state of health? and skin type? If you have a serious medical problem, such as diabetes, a heart disorder, hypertension, obesity, kidney dysfunction or other metabolic malfunction, or are on daily medication, consult with your health practitioner first.*

❊ *It is best to avoid extended periods of heat during pregnancy, especially in the early months.*

❊ *If you have exercised vigorously first, it may not be wise to risk further water loss.*

❊ *Novices should limit exposure in saunas to 6 minutes or less, and veterans to no more than 15 minutes. Get out immediately if you begin to feel faint or nauseous.*

Afterwards, shower and shampoo thoroughly to remove residual salts, acids, metals or chemicals. Moisturise your skin and drink plenty of water to replace lost fluids. Never drink alcohol during or after a sauna, as it has a dehydrating effect on the body.

# Essential Oils to Use

Apart from their obvious therapeutic effects, some essential oils have definite aphrodisiac properties. These exotic and captivating oils can enhance a romantic interlude with someone special in a jacuzzi. The following blend is ideal for such an occasion, and will promote a mood of relaxation and togetherness. Add oils drop by drop in the following proportions until the water is sufficiently scented, but not overpowering.

*2 drops rose essential oil*
*2 drops geranium essential oil*
*1 drop clary sage essential oil*

Or perhaps you would prefer a blend that will nourish, moisturise and soften the skin as well.

*35 ml (1 fl oz) almond oil*
*15 ml (½ fl oz) hazelnut oil*
*5 ml (⅙ fl oz) jojoba oil*
*5 ml (⅙ fl oz) wheat germ oil*
*10 drops rose essential oil*
*10 drops geranium essential oil*
*5 drops clary sage essential oil*

Thoroughly blend all the oils together and store in an airtight, amber-coloured glass bottle. Add 10 drops of the oil blend, or more if preferred, a drop at a time, until the water is sufficiently scented.

## Therapeutic Blends

Use any of the following essential oils in the jacuzzi, either singly or in combination, to suit your particular needs.

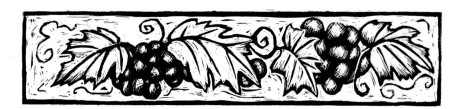

| ESSENTIAL OIL | BENEFICIAL EFFECT |
|---|---|
| BASIL | *Refreshing, uplifting, stimulating and invigorating. Especially good for anxiety and headaches.* |
| BAY LEAF | *Very aromatic; soothing to the senses and comforting to tired and aching limbs.* |
| BERGAMOT | *Aromatic, antiseptic, refreshing, relaxing and uplifting. An inducement to restful sleep.* |
| CYPRESS | *Refreshing, stimulating and invigorating.* |
| EUCALYPTUS | *Highly aromatic; refreshing, head clearing (clears a stuffy nose to help you breathe more easily), and relieves muscular pain. Excellent in a sauna.* |
| GERANIUM (ALL TYPES) | *Very aromatic, refreshing and relaxing.* |
| JASMINE | *Soothing and relaxing; use in moderation as it has a powerful and heady fragrance.* |
| LAVENDER | *Refreshing, aromatic scent. Relaxing, calming and a natural disinfectant; benefits all skin types and is good for headaches, aching muscles, muscular pain, circulation, insomnia and cell renewal.* |
| LEMONGRASS | *Refreshing, stimulating and invigorating. Ideal for acne and oily skin; benefits the circulation and muscle tone.* |
| LOVAGE | *Relaxing and rejuvenating, with natural deodorising properties.* |
| MARJORAM | *Aromatic; calming, warming and fortifying; relieves tension, insomnia, headaches, muscular cramps and respiratory problems.* |
| NEROLI | *Very relaxing and excellent for the skin. Use sparingly as it has a very powerful scent. Expensive to buy.* |
| ORANGE | *Refreshing, reviving and restoring.* |
| PEPPERMINT | *Extra invigorating, comforting, satisfying. A refreshing scent that clears the head and improves breathing. Ideal for skin problems. However, use only in low concentration as it can easily irritate the skin, especially on sensitive areas.* |
| PINE | *Extra invigorating with a clean, refreshing scent; reviving, cleansing and stimulating. Excellent for sinus problems and 'flu.* |
| ROSE | *Relaxing and calming; softens the skin. One of the least toxic oils — good for children.* |
| ROSEMARY | *Refreshing aromatic scent, stimulating and invigorating; relieves stiff joints and aching muscles; good for fatigue and circulation.* |
| ROSEWOOD | *Uplifting, stimulating and invigorating.* |

| | |
|---|---|
| SAGE | *Aromatic; refreshing, relaxing and enlivening; reduces fatigue, clears sluggish skin and firms tissue. Quite toxic — use in moderation and do not use if breast-feeding. Clary sage is also comforting and satisfying, and reputed to be an aphrodisiac.* |
| SANDALWOOD | *Relaxing and uplifting; softens dry skin and is mildly astringent for oily skin.* |
| TANGERINE | *Stimulating and invigorating; helps to improve energy levels.* |
| TEA TREE | *Powerful antiseptic and fungicide. Highly disinfectant without being toxic; use for respiratory problems (head clearing for colds and 'flu), skin infections and wounds.* |
| YLANG-YLANG | *Calming, antiseptic, antidepressant, comforting and satisfying; use for anxiety, insomnia and frustration; regulates circulation. This oil has an extremely heady and strong scent and must be used sparingly. Too much can cause headaches.* |

## Inhalation

This method is particularly useful for colds, headaches, blocked sinuses, coughs and sore throats. Add 10 drops of essential oil to a handkerchief or tissue, and inhale the scent whenever needed. The handkerchief can also be placed beside the pillow at night to facilitate easier breathing. Alternatively, add a few drops of the appropriate oil to a bowl of boiling water and inhale the fumes.

Steaming offers an effective and direct method of treating respiratory and sinus problems. Oils which are ideal for vaporising are peppermint, eucalyptus and tea tree. Peppermint and eucalyptus contain menthol and eucalyptol respectively, and both have a cooling effect on the tissues and tired muscles. Other oils will help to smooth out that 'crumpled look' that dry skin can get, and restore tone to facial muscles.

The action of steam is twofold, internal as well as external. Essences in the vapour are absorbed through the delicate membrane of the nasal passages as well as through exposed skin, in the same way as occurs during a facial massage. This type of treatment is especially effective and beneficial in dealing with skin complaints such as acne, a condition that requires scrupulous deep cleansing to effect a cure.

To make your own vaporiser, half-fill a ceramic bowl with boiling water and add 5 drops of oil. Hold your face about 30 cm (12 in) away and cover your head with a towel large enough to form a tent; do not allow the vapour to escape. You should not steam your face for any longer than 10 minutes.

People with overly sensitive skin, dilated red veins, or who suffer from heart problems, breathing difficulties or asthma should consult their health practitioner before using an inhalation.

## FOR COLDS AND 'FLU

*2 drops eucalyptus essential oil*
*2 drops rosemary essential oil*
*1 drop lavender essential oil*
*or*
*2 drops tea tree essential oil*
*2 drops sandalwood essential oil*
*1 drop eucalyptus essential oil*

## FOR SINUSITIS

*2 drops each of*
*peppermint, eucalyptus and rosemary*
*essential oils*
*or 2 drops each of*
*basil, eucalyptus, lavender and*
*peppermint essential oils*

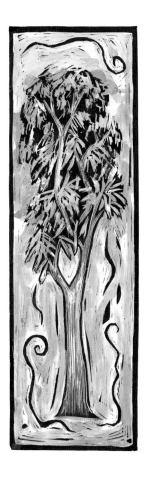

## FOR ACNE

Use this facial steam blend 3 to 4 times a week if acne is severe. Reduce to once a week when the condition begins to improve.

*1 drop lavender essential oil*
*1 drop chamomile essential oil*
*1 drop neroli essential oil*

Wait until the water has cooled to hand-hot temperature (about 38°C/100°F) before inhaling.

## FOR INSOMNIA

Just place one drop of lavender oil on your pillow, and you will be asleep in minutes. You can also try basil, chamomile, clary sage, juniper, neroli or sandalwood.

## FOR LABOURED BREATHING

Put a few drops of peppermint or eucalyptus oil on your handkerchief and inhale.

## FOR TRAVEL SICKNESS

Put a few drops of peppermint or lavender oil on a handkerchief or tissue and inhale.

## FOR MENTAL FATIGUE

When your concentration is flagging, you will find that inhaling a few drops of basil and bergamot oils on a handkerchief will conquer mental fatigue.

## WHEN DRIVING

To keep your head clear and concentration focused, add a few drops of basil oil to a handkerchief and inhale as needed. However, essential oils are not a cure for driver fatigue. If you are tired, rest until you are able to drive your car with safety.

# *Compresses*

An aromatic compress is made by soaking a piece of cotton gauze or a handkerchief in a bowl of hot water, to which the appropriate essential oil has been added. Compresses provide their beneficial effects by drawing new blood and lymph to the affected area, and absorbing any toxins. This method is therefore ideal for treating bruises, wounds and sprains, chest pain and skin problems.

To make a compress add 10 drops of the appropriate essential oil to 100 ml (3½ fl oz) of water. (The water can be either hot or cold, depending upon your needs.) The compress should be kept on the affected area for at least 2 hours.

Soak the piece of cloth in the liquid, then remove it and squeeze it gently until it stops dripping. Apply the compress to the affected area and cover with plastic wrap. To increase its ability to retain heat and to effect absorption through the skin, wrap the compress with a prewarmed towel, then place a blanket over the towel and patient.

Hot compresses may be used to soothe old injuries, sprains, muscular aches and pains, neuralgia, painful periods and skin problems. A cold compress is used to treat recent sprains, bruises or swellings, and headaches. Cold compresses are far more effective if they are refrigerated first.

A number of common problems can be treated effectively with compresses made with the following essential oils:

BRUISES AND BUMPS • *Lavender, hyssop, calendula, rosemary or geranium.*

CHILBLAINS • *Lavender, lemon, rosemary, camphor, geranium or ginger.*

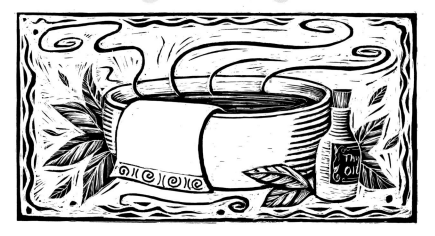

CRAMP • *Basil, cypress, geranium, ginger or marjoram.*

DRY, FLAKY SKIN • *Lavender.*

ECZEMA, DRY • *Chamomile, lavender or geranium.*

ECZEMA, WEEPING • *Bergamot or juniper.*

FEVERS • *Lavender, eucalyptus, melissa, peppermint and chamomile.*

GRAZES, CUTS AND MINOR WOUNDS • *Lavender, eucalyptus or thyme. For infected wounds use tea tree, chamomile, lavender, eucalyptus or thyme.*

HEADACHES • *Lavender, chamomile, marjoram and peppermint. Relieve tension headaches by putting a few drops of lavender oil in a bowl of warm water, soak a handkerchief in it and wring out, then apply to the back of the neck.*

INSECT BITES • *Lavender, chamomile, eucalyptus, melissa or thyme.*

ITCHY SKIN • *Chamomile.*

MUSCLES, STIFF AND ACHING • *Rosemary, thyme, lavender and eucalyptus.*

NEURALGIA • *Chamomile and geranium.*

PRICKLY HEAT • *Chamomile, geranium and lavender.*

PSORIASIS • *Bergamot and lavender.*

RASH • *Lavender and chamomile.*

RHEUMATISM • *Rosemary, oregano and thyme.*

SPRAINS AND STRAINS • *Eucalyptus, lavender, thyme and chamomile.*

SUNBURN • *Lavender and chamomile.*

# Vaporisation

Essential oils can be used to perfume or disinfect a room in a number of different ways. They can remove stale and unwanted odours, add a pleasurable fragrance to a bedroom or create a special atmosphere, make a house seem inviting to guests or freshen a sick room, and kill airborne viruses and prevent bacteria from spreading.

Try the following ideas to give your surroundings a fragrant air:

✳ *Add a few drops of essential oil to a shallow dish of warm water set on a sunny windowsill, or near a radiator. A few drops of rosewood oil is an ideal way to refresh a stuffy room.*

✳ *Moisten a sponge with boiling water and add a few drops of essential oil. Place the sponge in a dish in the bathroom or a sick room, and moisten it with boiling water twice a day. Refresh the sponge with a few extra drops of oil twice a week. Use lavender or peppermint oil in a sick room as additional protection against bacteria.*

✳ *Help to revitalise your body and restore health after illness by adding tangerine oil to your bath; or, take it as an inhalation.*

✳ *Placing a few drops of oil on a warm light bulb will quickly fill a room with fragrance. Do not use oils containing alcohol and only use light bulbs rated at least 45 watts for maximum effect.*

✳ *Burning essential oils will kill airborne bacteria and fungi. Try thyme, lavender, pine or eucalyptus for their fresh fragrance and disinfectant qualities. For instance, if you have an open fire, scatter a few drops on the wood before stoking. Or, add a few drops to a candlewick before lighting.*

✳ *Burning oil in a simmering pot will gently disperse the fragrant vapour. A simmering pot is a small ceramic vessel which is open at the top, and has a ceramic saucer that sits over this opening. A small candle inside the vessel provides the necessary heat. To use your oil burner, add about 10 drops of your chosen oil to 1 cup (155 ml/5 fl oz) of boiling water. Preheat the saucer by lighting the candle underneath, and then three-quarters fill it with the fragrant water, topping up as required.*

✳ *Terracotta scent pots are another delightful way to perfume rooms or cupboards with your favourite essential oil. Hang the empty pot in an appropriate place (the clothes rail in your wardrobe is perfect), and add 6 drops of oil to start, then 1 to 2 drops every week. The terracotta holds the fragrance and gently releases it into the air. Simmering pots and terracotta scent pots are both available from herb, craft and gift shops.*

✳ *In a sauna add 2 drops of pine or eucalyptus oil to a ladle of water, or 15 drops to a small bucket of water, for a very pleasant inhalation with an antiseptic effect.*

✳ *Sprinkle a few drops of essential oil on a tissue and place it in the air vent of your car; this will keep it smelling fragrant and fresh as you drive. Citrus oils will refresh stale air, while basil and peppermint will help you to remain alert.*

✳ *Long hours of study are taxing to both the mind and body. To help you cope and remain alert, add a drop of essential oil to a page in each book that you are using. Try any of the following:*

BASIL     *To clear your head.*

BERGAMOT     *To bring freshness.*

CARDAMOM     *For reducing mental fatigue.*

LAVENDER     *For physical and mental tension.*

ROSE     *To lift your spirits.*

TANGERINE     *To increase energy levels.*

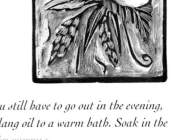

✳ *To counter stress, add a few drops of essential oil to your bath water. Choose from lavender, sandalwood, ylang-ylang and rose. A mixture of lavender and rosewood in an evening bath is a great way to unwind.*

✳ *To lift depressing moods, add the following essential oils to your bath water:*

MELANCHOLY • *Rose, neroli or chamomile.*

ANXIETY • *Chamomile, neroli or lavender.*

ANGER • *Rose or chamomile.*

✳ *Revitalise yourself after a busy day, when you still have to go out in the evening, by adding a few drops of bergamot and ylang-ylang oil to a warm bath. Soak in the water for 10 minutes, breathing in the restorative vapours.*

✳ *To create a particular mood, essential oils can be added to a pump-spray bottle with a fine mist setting and simply sprayed into the air. Choose from any of the following oils to create that special atmosphere:*

| | |
|---|---|
| ROSE, JASMINE AND YLANG-YLANG | *Romantic, lazy and warm; use in small amounts.* |
| CINNAMON, ORANGE AND CLOVE | *Spicy and warm.* |
| FRANKINCENSE AND MYRRH | *Festive.* |
| PATCHOULI | *Cosy.* |
| ROSEWOOD | *Reassuring.* |
| SANDALWOOD | *Relaxing and exotic; encourages conversation.* |
| YLANG-YLANG | *Exotic.* |

These oils are only a basic guide and should not be the limit of your imagination or experimentation. Learn to choose your own oils, and experiment with different blends according to your personal taste.

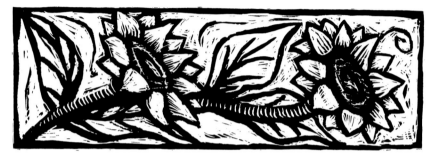

## AIR PURIFICATION SPRAY

This is a very strong antiseptic spray. Use in a sick room and it will help to combat the spread of germs throughout the house.

*25 drops lemon essential oil*
*25 drops lavender essential oil*
*15 drops thyme essential oil*
*15 drops clove essential oil*
*10 drops tea tree essential oil*
*5 drops peppermint essential oil*
*5 drops eucalyptus essential oil*
*50 ml (2 fl oz) vodka*
*500 ml (16 fl oz) distilled water*

Blend the oils together, then dissolve the essential oils in the vodka and blend thoroughly with the distilled water. Store in a pump-spray bottle and use on a fine mist setting, as required.

## ROOM FRESHENER SPRAY

Use this to eliminate household odours, or whenever an antiseptic or disinfectant spray is needed.

Choose from any of the following oils, listed in descending order of their antiseptic powers: thyme, orange flower, bergamot, juniper, clove, lavender, niaouli, peppermint, rosemary, sandalwood or eucalyptus.

*30 drops essential oil of choice*
*5 ml (⅙ fl oz) vodka*
*500 ml (16 fl oz) distilled water*

Prepare as for *Air Purification Spray* (see page 22).

# *Internal Use*

It is important to realise that essential oils are extremely strong and powerful. In some circumstances, just 1 teaspoon (5 ml/⅙ fl oz) of a particular oil taken internally may prove to be lethal. For this reason they should only be taken under the direction of your health practitioner, or following advice from an individual trained in the use of essential oils.

Some of the edible oils, such as lemon, can be used in minute amounts with safety. Again, before use, discuss your individual circumstances with your health practitioner. This fact cannot be emphasised strongly enough.

## FLAVOURED TEAS

Teas can be flavoured by adding 5 drops of essential oil to a packet of regular tea leaves. Alternatively, place 1 drop of oil on a tea bag and use this to make a whole pot of tea. Citrus oil is especially appropriate. It is ideal for treating coughs and colds, headaches, indigestion and constipation. Another idea is to dissolve a teaspoon of honey in a glass of warm water and then add 1 to 3 drops of the essential oil — again, lemon is perfect.

Take one glass or cup 2 to 3 times daily.

# CHAPTER TWO

# Oils to Make and Keep

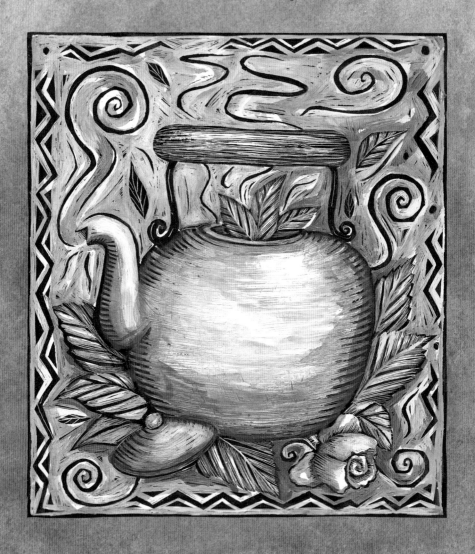

# The Life Force of Plants

The 'life force' of a herb or flower is contained in its essential oil. It is this substance that gives plants their distinctive aroma along with many unique health and beauty care applications. Most flowers, leaves, seeds, grains, roots and wood resins contain essential oils, usually in minute quantities. Quite often, it is the smallest flowers which are the most intensely perfumed. Other plants, such as the orange tree, provide several different volatile oils: the oil from the fruit is called orange, that from the leaves is called petitgrain, and the flowers yield that wonderful fragrance known as neroli.

Essential oils vary in the intensity of their colour and quality. Some are very pale pastel shades, almost colourless, such as basil, which is light green, and chamomile, which has a bluish tinge. Other oils are deeply pigmented, such as rose which is orange-red, and patchouli, which is dark brown.

Unlike vegetable oils, the odoriferous molecules contained in essential oils tend to be extremely volatile; this means they evaporate quickly, especially when they are warmed. With the exception of garlic and cinnamon, essential oils are lighter than water and are usually quite fluid. However, some do have a viscous consistency, rather like honey.

Pure essential oils can be obtained through distillation, enfleurage, maceration, dissolving and pressing by hand. Choosing the appropriate method is important, for it will affect the oil's quality and particular therapeutic properties.

## Distillation

In this method, steam is passed over the leaves or flowers and the essential oil vaporises in the steam. It is then cooled so that it condenses, for ease of collection.

## Enfleurage

Flowers are first spread out in a glass dish containing purified fat. They are left for up to 72 hours, during which time their aromatic scent will soak into the fat. Exhausted blooms are replaced with fresh ones until the fat is completely saturated with essential oil. This fragrant fat is then soaked in alcohol until all the essential oil has been dissolved into it. The resulting liquid is then gently heated, thus evaporating the alcohol and leaving the essential oil intact.

This method of extraction is beyond the capabilities of most people. However, a simple variation using either salt or a base oil, described later in this chapter, is just as effective.

## Maceration

This method is similar to enfleurage, except that it utilises a vegetable oil to extract the essential oil. Vegetable oils impregnated in this way are suitable for massage or cosmetic applications.

## Dissolving

In some instances, solvents such as alcohol or ether are used to obtain essential oils. This particularly applies to the extraction of gums and resins, such as galbanum and myrrh, which use alcohol. Ether is more often used to obtain the essential oil from fresh plants and flowers. Following the application of the solvent it is then evaporated, leaving the valuable essential oil behind.

## Pressing by Hand

Oils from members of the citrus family, such as oranges, limes, lemons and bergamots, are extracted by this method. The rinds are squeezed by hand until the oil glands burst, thus releasing the essential oil.

You can employ this method quite easily. Next time you are eating an orange do not discard the peel with its precious oil, which is good for both the face and body. Instead, scratch the outer surface with a sharp pointed object, then squeeze the peel until you see the oil coming out. Gently rub the scoured peel directly onto your face or body to obtain its benefits as a skin tonic and exfoliant.

# Extraction of Oils at Home

Pure essential oils can be easily extracted at home without the need for elaborate equipment. Alternatively, methods similar to the commercial ones previously discussed can be employed, using a carrier oil or alcohol to extract the volatile essences.

## Sun Distillation

Most sweet-scented flowers, herbs and fruits will yield their aromatic oils by this process.

Place fresh flower petals or herbs in a large, wide-mouthed glass jar, and cover with distilled water. If you are working with fruit, such as citrus, squeeze the rinds so that the oil glands burst. Seal the jar with plastic clingwrap so that it is airtight, and leave it where it will receive plenty of hot sun every day.

When a thin film of oil appears on the top of the water, gently lift it off with cottonwool and squeeze it into a small glass bottle. Reseal the distilling jar. Repeat the process until no more oil appears.

## Kettle Distillation

This process requires no elaborate equipment, yet it is still an effective method for producing small quantities of essential oil.

You will need a large, old-fashioned kettle, preferably one made from enamel or stainless steel, that is boiled on the stove. In addition, you will require a length of rubber hose (approximately 1 metre/3 feet), a short length of glass tubing, a large shallow basin, and a collection flask, such as a glass jar.

Place 500 g (16 oz) of fresh flower petals or herbs in the kettle. Add sufficient distilled water to fill the kettle to half-way. Replace the lid and seal the edges with plasticine to prevent steam from escaping. Cut the rubber hose in two, so that one length is three times longer than the other. Insert the glass tube between the two lengths of hose, attaching the shortest end to the spout of the kettle.

Put the kettle on the stove over a low heat. Place the basin so that it is higher than the kettle and fill it with ice-cold water and ice cubes. Run the hose through the water, letting the longer end hang down into the collection flask.

Let the water in the kettle simmer until it has completely evaporated. The glass tube will allow you to observe this process, so that you will see when no more steam is passing through. Throughout the process, keep the basin topped up with iced water or ice cubes.

In the collection flask two layers will then be seen; being the distilled water with the pure essence floating on top of it. Gently lift the essence with cottonwool and squeeze it into a small, amber-coloured glass bottle.

## Steam Distillation

This process is slightly more complicated than the simple 'kettle still' described above. However, the necessary equipment can be purchased from a scientific supplier and, if you are serious about producing your own essential oils, this method will enable you to process a larger quantity of plant material, thus obtaining far more essential oil.

As well as providing the essence to be collected, an additional benefit is obtained by steam distillation. The water remaining in the still will also contain a small portion of the herb or flower scent, giving you a floral water of commercial standards.

To make a 'steam still', you will need a distilling flask, a tripod, a heat source (such as a gas burner), two clamps, a condensing tube with two hoses attached (to let the water in and out), and a receiving flask (to collect the oil) attached to the end of the condensor. Place the distilling flask on the tripod, with one clamp attached to the top of the flask to hold it in place. Put the heat source under the tripod. Fix the condensor horizontally in the other clamp, with one end attached to the distilling flask, and the other end inserted into the receiving flask. The two hoses should be inserted into the nozzles on either side of the condensor, with the water entering the condensor through the hose closest to the receiving flask, and water exiting the condensor through the hose closest to the distilling flask.

## STEAM DISTILLATION

Two-thirds fill the distillation flask with rainwater or distilled water and add about 500 g (16 oz) of fresh herbs or flowers. Bring to a gentle boil. The liquid should now be steaming in the distillation flask and slowly condensing in the cooling condenser. Turn off the heat when the oil has been collected. The amount of essence collected will only be minute: for example, 500 g (16 oz) of orange blossoms only produces 0.5 g of essential oil.

The following list gives the yield proportion of different herbs and flowers:

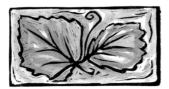

EUCALYPTUS • *500 g (16 oz) will yield 2.5 g*
GERANIUM • *500 g (16 oz) will yield 0.5 g*
LAVENDER • *500 g (16 oz) will yield 2.5 g*
MINT • *500 g (16 oz) will yield 0.575 g*
ROSE PETALS • *500 g (16 oz) will yield 0.02 g*

## *Preparation*

Before commencing the distillation process, note:

&#10042; *Dry and hard or fibrous substances should be bruised or macerated in water before distilling.*

&#10042; *Salted flowers and herbs are superior to fresh ones, as they reach the full development of their aromatic properties in a shorter time. To salt flowers and herbs, spread them on a shallow, flat tray and sprinkle with a small quantity of salt. Place the salted material in a glass jar and cover with distilled water. Seal the jar and allow to stand overnight. Add the contents of the jar to your still, adjusting the amount of distilled water if necessary.*

&#10042; *Distilled essential oils may have a smoky odour at first. Exposing the oil to the air for a short time will remove this, after which the oil should be kept in a tightly sealed bottle.*

&#10042; *When distilling, ensure that the condensing tube is kept cold. The condensing steam must drip, not run.*

## *Enfleurage*

This process can be used to extract a pure essence, or to create an essence in a carrier oil, such as almond, sunflower, olive or any other seed oil. Although this method is not quite the same as the traditional commercial one, it is just as effective.

### PURE ESSENTIAL OIL

Pick fresh herbs or flower petals early in the morning after the dew has evaporated, as this is when they are at their most fragrant. Select only perfect specimens and discard any that are damaged. Make sure you keep the different types of herbs separate.

Place a layer of petals or herb leaves in the bottom of a small ceramic casserole or jar (never use glass or metal) and sprinkle a thin layer of coarse salt over them. Repeat this 'layering' procedure until the vessel is full. Put the lid on the casserole or jar, and seal tightly with plasticine. Leave it undisturbed for a month in a cool, dark cupboard.

After a month, strain the mixture through muslin cloth into a glass jar, squeezing all liquid from the herbs. Seal the jar and leave it where it will receive plenty of sunlight for 6 weeks. Any sediment will then settle. Decant the essential oil and store in small, amber-coloured glass bottles.

## FRAGRANT OILS

Although fragrant oils are not as strong as a pure essence, they are ideal for use as body and bath oils.

Spread fresh herbs or flower petals on a shallow, flat tray, and sprinkle a small quantity of non-iodised salt over them. Place a layer of these salted herbs in a wide-mouthed glass jar, followed by a layer of cottonwool which has been combed out thinly and soaked in a suitable carrier oil. Repeat this 'layering' procedure until the jar is full. Seal the jar with a piece of plastic clingwrap, and secure it with a rubber band. Leave the jar in a sunny spot for at least 15 days, then squeeze the fragrant oil from the whole mass. Strain it through muslin cloth and store in a bottle with a tight-fitting cap.

If the fragrance is not strong enough, repeat the procedure with a fresh batch of herbs or flowers, soaking the cottonwool in the existing fragrant oil.

## *Maceration*

This method is especially suitable for extracting the essential oil of roses, but it will work well for all aromatic flowers and herbs. Place the plant material in a stainless steel or enamel saucepan, cover with an odourless seed oil, such as apricot kernel oil or grapeseed oil, and heat to 65°C (150°F). Remove pan from heat and cool. Strain mixture and store in an airtight bottle.

## *Calendula Oil*

*Calendula officinalis,* commonly known as the 'pot marigold', is one of the finest natural antiseptics for cuts and all open wounds known to man. It is both healing and rejuvenating to the skin, and is excellent in the treatment of pimples. When rubbed into the feet calendula oil will relieve persistent soreness.

To extract this essential oil, tightly pack fresh *Calendula* flower heads into a wide-mouthed glass jar with an airtight lid and cap securely. Leave the jar in the sun for several days until an oily orange fluid appears on the bottom: this will be pure calendula oil.

## Citrus Oils

Citrus oils can be obtained by hand pressing, or through any of the distillation methods previously described. When pressing by hand the rinds are squeezed until the oil glands burst, thus releasing the oil. The minute droplets are then removed by gently scraping the oil into a suitable container.

# Combining and Blending Oils

Throughout this book, specific instructions are given for blending certain oils to suit particular needs. However, there is also plenty of scope for you to mix your own blends.

Mixing fragrant essential oils is an art in itself. At first no doubt you will find yourself mixing some curious blends! Trial and error, along with a sensitive nose, should give you the desired result. Some problems and people respond to more dilute solutions, while other circumstances will require a greater strength. Start with an average blend, or less, as your guideline and work from there. It is far easier to adjust a recipe by adding oils than to tone down an overly strong blend.

Massaging provides a good example of the uses of different blends of oils: you may find that a lower concentration gives the best results for emotional problems, whereas a higher concentration will often be more successful in dealing with physical complaints.

Do not assume that for oils to be effective they must always be combined with many other oils. Quite often a single oil will be sufficient for a particular need. When you do blend oils, do not use any more than three. More may quite easily confuse the body systems and cancel out any beneficial effect. There are, however, exceptions to this rule, and in these instances a recipe is provided.

The following table (see pages 32–33) will give you a basic idea as to which oils can be blended with each other. It is by no means 'carved in stone', but will, rather, provide a good starting point. Experimentation will enable you to explore further possibilities for particular applications.

| OIL | BLEND WITH |
|---|---|
| BASIL | *Bergamot, geranium, hyssop, neroli, marjoram, melissa and lavender.* |
| BERGAMOT | *Chamomile, coriander, cypress, geranium, jasmine, lemon, myrrh, rose and sandalwood.* |
| BLACK PEPPER | *Cypress, frankincense and sandalwood. All spice oils.* |
| CAMPHOR | *Frankincense and neroli.* |
| CHAMOMILE | *Bergamot, geranium, lavender, lemon, marjoram, neroli, rose and ylang-ylang.* |
| CLARY SAGE | *Bergamot, citrus oils, cypress, geranium, jasmine, juniper, lavender and sandalwood.* |
| CLOVE | *Basil, citrus and spice oils.* |
| CORIANDER | *Bergamot, cypress, lemon, neroli, orange and spice oils.* |
| CYPRESS | *Bergamot, clary sage, juniper, lavender, lemon, orange and sandalwood.* |
| EUCALYPTUS | *Hyssop, lavender, lemon, lemongrass, melissa, pine and rose.* |
| FRANKINCENSE | *All oils.* |
| GERANIUM (*PELARGONIUM* SPP.) | *All oils.* |
| GINGER | *Citrus and spice oils.* |
| HYSSOP | *Clary sage, lavender, rosemary, sage and citrus oils.* |
| JASMINE | *All oils.* |
| JUNIPER | *Bergamot, citrus oils, cypress, geranium, lavender, rosemary and sandalwood.* |

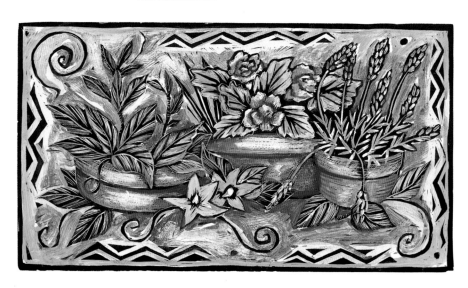

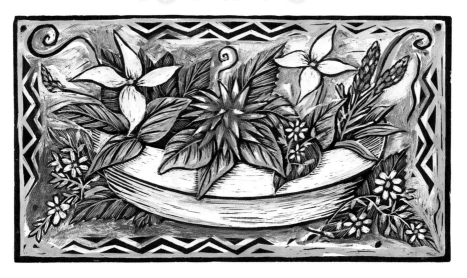

| | |
|---|---|
| LAVENDER | *Most oils.* |
| LEMON | *Chamomile, eucalyptus, frankincense, geranium, juniper, neroli and ylang-ylang.* |
| LEMONGRASS | *Basil, geranium, jasmine and lavender.* |
| MARJORAM (SWEET) | *Bergamot, chamomile, cypress, lavender and rosemary.* |
| MELISSA | *Geranium, juniper, neroli and ylang-ylang.* |
| MYRRH | *Camphor, lavender and spice oils.* |
| NEROLI | *Most oils.* |
| NIAOULI | *Lavender, pine and mint.* |
| PATCHOULI | *Basil, bergamot, geranium, juniper, lavender, myrrh, neroli, pine and rose.* |
| PEPPERMINT | *Black pepper, melissa, marjoram and spice oils. Only blend in small amounts with other oils.* |
| PINE | *Eucalyptus, lavender, rosemary, sage and spice oils.* |
| ROSE | *Most oils.* |
| ROSEMARY | *Basil, frankincense, lavender, lemon and peppermint.* |
| SAGE | *Bergamot, hyssop, lemon, lavender, melissa, peppermint and rosemary.* |
| SANDALWOOD | *Black pepper, cypress, frankincense, jasmine, lemon, myrrh, neroli and ylang-ylang.* |
| TANGERINE | *Frankincense, mandarin, myrrh, orange, pine and spice oils.* |
| TEA TREE | *Citrus oils, lavender, rosemary and spice oils.* |
| THYME | *Bergamot, citrus oils, melissa and rosemary.* |
| YLANG-YLANG | *Most oils.* |

# *Quantities to Use*

The following quantities are given only as a general guide, as every individual — and their needs — is different.

These are safe approximations and should not be exceeded, unless on the advice of a qualified practitioner. When administering oils to children, always halve the dosage as they are more sensitive to them than adults.

## *Massage*

An essential oil in its concentrated form can sting or burn if it is applied directly to the skin. It must first be diluted with a suitable carrier oil (see page 63); for preference, use one that is pure, unrefined and cold–pressed.

Remember that although carrier oils will readily penetrate the skin, they do become rancid when exposed to the air. This occurs even more rapidly with essential oil blends which will, therefore, only be at their best for no longer than two to three months. It is wise not to mix more oil than can be used within that time. In most circumstances, it would be prudent to mix oils only for immediate use.

When selecting essential oils for use in massage, first decide which condition you want to treat. Then put enough carrier oil in an eggcup or other suitable container, such as a medicine glass, and add the essential oil or oils. One full body massage uses between 10 to 20 ml (⅓ to ⅔ fl oz) of carrier oil, depending upon body size and skin type. Four to six drops of essential oil in the base oil will usually be sufficient. For a mixture of two or three oils add equal amounts, unless specified in a particular recipe.

An excellent massage blend can be made by adding between 15 to 30 drops of essential oil to 50 ml (2 fl oz) of carrier oil. This carrier oil is made up of 40 ml (1½ fl oz) of your chosen oil, 5 ml (⅙ fl oz) of wheat germ oil to extend the life of the blend, and 5 ml (⅙ fl oz) avocado oil for greater penetration.

If you have made up a blend such as this one, don't forget to store it in an amber-coloured glass bottle, away from direct sunlight and heat, and to label and date it.

## Baths

Aromatic baths are highly therapeutic, particularly for muscular aches and pains, skin disorders, circulation problems, tension, fatigue and insomnia.

Add 4 to 10 drops of your chosen oil or oils (unless other quantities are directed) to a bath of warm water after the water has settled, and mix it around with your hand. Relax in the water for about 10 minutes, closing any windows and doors for maximum effect. Finish off with an after-bath massage oil.

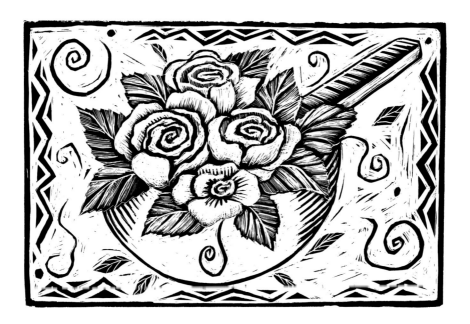

## Therapeutic Footbaths

Three to four drops of essential oil in a basin of hot water is usually sufficient. Add more if the mixture is not aromatic enough. Finish off with a therapeutic foot massage, using a fragrant oil.

# *Perfumes*

Many essential oils have an acceptable scent and, on their own, they are delightful to the nose. However you have enormous scope from the large range of both flower and herb oils now available to improve upon a basic fragrance, and make your own special blend.

When blending oils, there are three notes in scent to consider: top, middle and base. Top, of course, is the first to stimulate the olfactory nerves and it is the highest, sweetest and most uplifting scent. It is also the quickest to evaporate. Middle notes are more moderate or mellow, while base notes are heavy, lasting and the most lingering.

A balanced combination of the three will usually produce an acceptable and pleasing fragrance. Too much top will be overly intense, light and heady, whereas too much base will give a heavy, pungent aroma.

Spices will always blend with spices, fruits with fruits, and flowers with flowers. However, there is no need to restrict yourself to these combinations, since this would limit the potential of your perfume–making. Experimentation is the key to success, although at first you will more than likely end up with some very peculiar blends! Lemon and lavender are good neutralisers for any 'aroma disasters'.

In concentrated form essential oils can be extremely overpowering. To achieve a desirable perfume, the mixture must be diluted with alcohol; this will also preserve the scent of the oil or oil blends. Use either pure alcohol (if you can obtain it), vodka or a perfumer's alcohol that has been denatured. The latter is available as 'orrisroot tincture' by mail order from The Fragrant Garden, Portsmouth Road, Erina NSW 2250, Australia.

When blending oils, the following proportions apply:

Perfume 15 to 25% essential oils to 75 to 85% alcohol

Toilet Water 12 to 15% essential oils blended with 50 to 60% alcohol, with the balance made up of distilled water.

(See Chapter 3 for perfume and toilet water recipes.)

## *Storage*

Once you have either purchased or extracted your own essential oils it is important to ensure that they last as long as possible. Therefore, try to observe the following:

❋ *Store them in a cool place, away from strong light and heat. A cupboard (not in the kitchen or bathroom) is ideal.*

❋ *Use glass storage bottles that are dark (amber) coloured and airtight. Never use plastic — oils are very potent substances and will eventually eat their way through the plastic.*

❋ *Never keep mixed oils, especially those made with a carrier oil base, any longer than two months. They begin to oxidise as soon as they are blended.*

❋ *Keep your oils clearly labelled. Until you become an expert in distinguishing the various scents by smell alone, it is easy to get the bottles confused.*

❋ *Replace lids on bottles of essential oil immediately to maintain quality, as they are adversely affected by heat, light, oxygen and moisture. If properly kept, essential oils last for up to a year.*

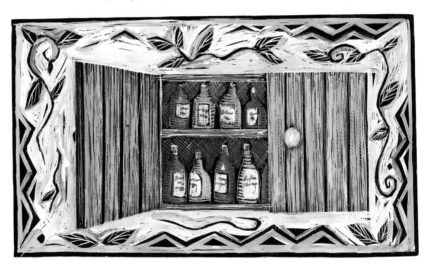

# A Guide to Essential Oils

Newcomers to the fragrant world of flowers and herbs could be forgiven for any confusion they may experience when they first encounter all the essential oils. There are so many and they all have so many uses and benefits, it must seem overwhelming, to say the least. At first it may, therefore, be difficult to determine which oils to start with.

The following essential oils will provide an excellent basic 'wardrobe' for most situations. As you become more familiar with the various herbs and flowers and their beneficial properties, you can add more.

CHAMOMILE

*Very soothing, relaxing, calming and comforting to the nerves; an inducement to sound natural sleep. It is the first choice for treating children's ailments, and can be used for teething troubles, in the bath to ease nerves and tetchiness, and to help in the treatment of red, inflamed eyes. For general first aid, chamomile can be used in the treatment of burns (including sunburn), skin ailments such as psoriasis and eczema, sprains and strains, bruises, rashes, wounds, infections and windburn.*

EUCALYPTUS

*Highly aromatic; refreshing, head–clearing (clears a stuffy nose to help you breathe more easily), and relieves muscular pain. Aids formation of skin tissue. Massage eucalyptus oil into feet as an inducement to deep sleep. Also makes an antiseptic air freshener. Its anti-inflammatory, antiseptic, antibiotic, deodorising and antiviral properties make eucalyptus oil a key addition to any basic kit of essential oils. In first aid situations, this oil is useful for animal bites, colds, grazes and cuts, infections, insect bites, itchy skin, over-exercised muscles, sunburn and prickly heat, swellings and windburn.*

GERANIUM

*Very aromatic, refreshing and relaxing. It is helpful in treating chilblains, blisters, muscle cramp, dry and flaky skin conditions and prickly heat. Use it to treat menstrual problems and as a highly aromatic, yet delightful, insect repellent.*

LAVENDER

*Refreshing aromatic scent; relaxing and calming, and a natural disinfectant, antibiotic and detoxifier. These natural attributes all contribute to the healing process and prevent scarring of the skin tissue. An excellent first aid remedy for insect bites and small burns. Its low toxicity makes it a good oil to use with children's injuries. Use it also for animal bites, bruises, bumps, burns, dry and flaky skin, as a facial cleanser, to clear blemished skin, grazes and cuts, infections, insect bites, as an insect repellent, and for prickly heat, rashes, sprains and strains, swellings, wounds, muscular pain, headaches and windburn.*

*Face cleanser — Mix 1 drop of oil to 100 ml (3½ fl oz) of distilled water and apply with a cotton ball. Do not use on oily or spotted skin.*

*Blemished skin — Mix 2 drops each of lavender oil and chamomile oil in the palm of your hands, then massage into facial skin each evening after cleansing thoroughly. Leave on overnight.*

*If a blemish is coming up, dab on 1 drop of lavender oil to help it disappear.*

PEPPERMINT · *Extra invigorating, comforting, and satisfying. A refreshing scent that clears the head and improves breathing. It is a natural antiseptic and pain reliever, and can be used in the treatment of colds and 'flu, headaches, travel sickness, sunburn, toothache, indigestion and summer itch, and as an insect repellent. Use in low concentrations (no more than 1%) on inflamed or sensitive skin. High concentrations have a tendency to sting and burn the skin.*

ROSEMARY · *Refreshing aromatic scent, stimulating and invigorating; relieves stiff joints and aching muscles and is the perfect bath oil after a long tiring day. It is an antiseptic oil that can be used as an insect repellent, to encourage hair growth and to help control dandruff, aid the circulation, help relieve fatigue and headaches (including migraine), and to treat muscular sprains, arthritis and rheumatism.*

TEA TREE · *Toning and head clearing. Highly disinfectant without being toxic. This oil is a powerful antiseptic and fungicide that can be used to treat wounds, minor cuts and abrasions, skin infections, acne, bites and stings, temporary relief of nasal and chest congestion, candida, athlete's foot, toothache, pyorrhoea (gum disease) and sunburn. Use it as a facial cleanser for oily or spotted skin. Mix 1 drop of oil to 100 ml (3½ fl oz) of distilled water and apply with a cotton ball.*

THYME (ALL TYPES) · *Delightful aromatic scent; a natural antiseptic and deodorant. The powerful antiviral properties of this oil make it a vital component in any basic kit of essential oils. Its active ingredient is thymol and as overuse can stimulate the thyroid gland and lymphatic system, it should be used in moderation and is not suitable for children (unless otherwise directed by your health practitioner). Never apply to the skin undiluted — blend it with an appropriate carrier oil first. Two or three drops to 5 ml (⅛ fl oz) of carrier oil should be sufficient.*
*This oil is especially useful for burning or including in an air freshener spray when colds and 'flu are around. It is also useful as an antiseptic and insect repellent, and to treat colds and respiratory problems, muscular pain, sprains and strains, and insect bites.*

Once you become more familiar with essential oils and their many uses, you can extend your 'basic wardrobe'. The following list is by no means exhaustive, but will allow you far more flexibility.

| OIL | PROPERTIES | USE TO TREAT |
|---|---|---|
| BASIL | Refreshing, uplifting, stimulating and invigorating. | Anxiety, concentration, headaches, respiratory problems. |
| BAY | Very aromatic; soothing to the senses and comforting to tired and aching limbs. | Sprains, aching limbs, rheumatism, colds and 'flu. |
| BERGAMOT | Aromatic; antiseptic, refreshing, relaxing and uplifting. | Anxiety; depression; aids digestion and appetite; an inducement to restful sleep. |
| BLACK PEPPER | Light, stimulating and soothing. | Stimulates circulation. Use for muscular aches and pains, rheumatism, colds and 'flu, and coughs. |
| CAMPHOR | Cooling, highly stimulating. | Oily skin, acne, coughs, cold, fevers, respiratory problems, arthritis, and rheumatism. Apply immediately to bruises and sprains as a cold compress to reduce swelling. |
| CINNAMON | Warming, astringent, antiseptic. | Digestion, coughs, colds and 'flu, exhaustion and viral infections. |
| CLARY SAGE | Warming and soothing. | Menstruation, dry skin, insect bites, sore throat, aches and pains, digestion and depression. Warning: Use sparingly — intoxication and headaches may result from overuse. |
| CLOVE | Warming, antiseptic, disinfectant, pain reliever. | Neuralgia, toothache, mouth and skin sores, flatulence, general debility, diarrhoea and infections. An excellent oil to use singly, or in combination in an air freshener spray. |

| | | |
|---|---|---|
| CORIANDER | Sweet, uplifting. | Digestion, nervous debility, flatulence, fatigue, rheumatic pain and 'flu. |
| CYPRESS | Refreshing, stimulating and invigorating. | Muscular cramps, 'flu, circulation, rheumatism and menopausal problems. |
| FRANKINCENSE | Warming, relaxing, tonic. | Ageing skin, inflammation, wounds, sores, stress and tension, nervous conditions and respiratory problems. |
| GINGER | Stimulating, tonic. | Loss of appetite, digestion, rheumatic and muscular aches and pains, nausea, colds, sore throat and diarrhoea. Invaluable as a bath oil for warding off colds. |
| HYSSOP | Sedative, decongestant. | Fades bruises and relieves stiffness from overwork or sport; arthritis, rheumatism, viral infections, circulatory and respiratory problems, anxiety and hypertension. Warning: Can be toxic and a danger to epileptics. |

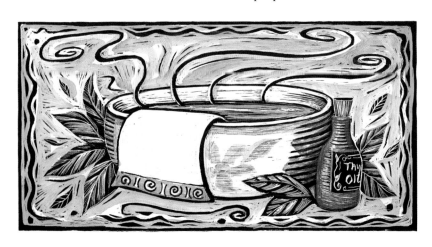

| | | |
|---|---|---|
| JUNIPER | Refreshing, stimulating, and invigorating. Natural disinfectant. | Aching muscles, skinsores, eczema, rheumatism, depression, obesity, urinary infections and respiratory problems. Warning: Do not use during pregnancy. |
| LEMON | Refreshing, invigorating and stimulating. Antiseptic. | Sore throats, digestive and respiratory problems, debility, circulation, oily skin, broken capillaries, fever, conditions. When used as an antiseptic, a 2% solution in distilled water stops small cuts bleeding. |
| LEMONGRASS | Refreshing, reviving and uplifting; healing for skin complaints. Antiseptic. | Muscle tone, acne, oily skin, infections, sore throats, digestion, insect repellent, headaches, circulation and respiratory problems. |
| MARJORAM (SWEET) | Aromatic; calming, warming and fortifying. | Colds, headaches, muscular cramps, tension, insomnia, sprains, bruises, rheumatism, anxiety, menstrual problems, circulatory disorders, digestion and respiratory problems. |
| MELISSA (LEMON BALM) | Delicious lemon scent; antidepressant; very relaxing and refreshing. | Neuralgia, tension, digestion, nervousness, fungal and bacterial infections, eczema, fevers, painful menstrual and respiratory problems, and diarrhoea. |
| MYRRH | Antiseptic, healing. | Loss of appetite; skin inflammations, candida, dermatitis, bacterial and fungal infections, wounds; catarrh and bronchitis. |
| NEROLI | Antiseptic; very relaxing, a heady scent. | Anxiety, nervous tension, depression, insomnia, diarrhoea, menopausal problems and skin rejuvenation. |

| | | |
|---|---|---|
| NIAOULI | Antiseptic, soothing and disinfectant. | Acne, skin ulcers, cuts and wounds, rheumatism, infections, burns, colds, and respiratory problems. |
| PATCHOULI | Exotic perfume; very relaxing and comforting; antiseptic and soothing. Antidepressant. | Anxiety; dry and mature skin, acne, eczema, skin inflammations, fungal infections and dandruff. |
| PINE | Extra invigorating with a clean, refreshing scent; reviving and stimulating. Antiseptic. Disinfectant. | Respiratory problems, asthma, sinus, colds and 'flu, catarrh, sore throats, chest infections, and muscular aches and pains. |
| ROSE | Relaxing and calming; softens the skin. Antiseptic; astringent. | Stress, headaches; suitable for all skin types; circulation and digestion. |
| SAGE | Aromatic; refreshing, relaxing and enlivening. Soothing. Antiseptic. | Fatigue; to clear sluggish skin and firm tissue. Warning: Quite toxic. Use in moderation and avoid completely if breastfeeding. |
| SANDALWOOD | Relaxing and calming. | Fatigue, nausea, acne, skin infections, fungal and bacterial infections, and respiratory problems. Will soften dry skin and act as a mild astringent on oily skin. |
| TANGERINE | Stimulating and invigorating. | Rheumatism, cellulite and stretch marks. Suitable for all skin types and for during pregnancy. Helps to improve energy levels, and is great as a pick-me-up after an illness. |
| YLANG-YLANG | Calming, comforting and satisfying. Antiseptic. | Anxiety, frustration, depression and insomnia. Regulates circulation and acts as a general tonic and sedative. |

# CHAPTER THREE

# Scentsational!

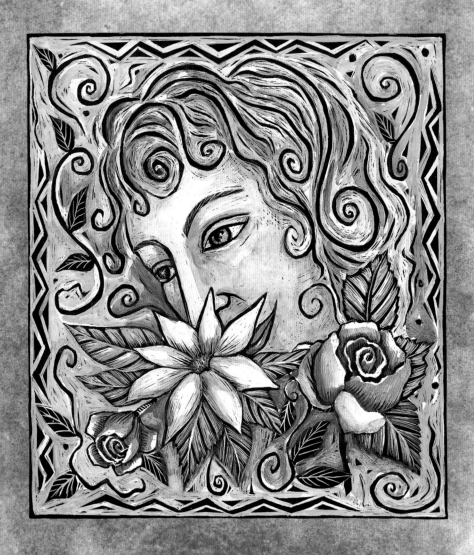

In every waking hour of every day, our olfactory nerves are invaded by many different smells. Some of these we find 'scentsational', while others are quite offensive.

When essences come in contact with the skin, they react according to an individual's body chemistry. It is this chemistry that makes us either alluring or an aromatic disaster. Over the centuries, perfumers have turned the blending of different essences into a passionate art form of finding that elusive scent which fulfils our fantasies.

With a little effort and practice, you will be able to make acceptable scents too. Whether they drive your partner wild with desire will depend upon your ability to refine your techniques! You may not create another 'Shalimar' by Guerlain or 'Opium' by Yves St Laurent, but it is possible to end up with some very exciting results.

## *How Do We Smell?*

The way in which we smell is an intricate process that involves our whole body system. It is not just a simple matter of the nose taking a sniff and sending an appropriate signal to the brain. This is only the starting point: from the brain, responses are triggered in the body's organs and fluids.

We are able to smell and to distinguish different scents through tiny filaments known as *olfactory hairs*, which are located in the top of the nose. These hairs catch odour molecules in the mucous membrane, which in turn affect the nerve cells and send signals to the brain.

We do not have anywhere near the number of olfactory hairs found in many animals. However, our sensitivity to smell is still quite considerable, enabling us to easily identify, remember and associate certain events with particular scents.

The nerve endings of the olfactory cells are very sensitive and so can be overcome by a particularly strong smell. Oils such as ylang-ylang and jasmine can definitely have an overpowering effect. They might be pleasant and enjoyable in small amounts, but large quantities can leave you feeling light-headed, and with a sickening headache.

Through our olfactory cells, we may enjoy the many delightful fragrances that pervade our life. Our ability to smell can transport us back in time, tapping into our emotions and memories in a way no other sense can.

## Smell, Feeling and Memory

No other sense — neither taste, sight nor hearing — can tap our memories or emotions as directly as our sense of smell. It is a key part of that first instinct we experience when we meet a person and either like or dislike them, without really knowing why. This 'reason why' is usually simple: subconsciously, we do not like the way they smell. By the same token, we are automatically attracted to someone whose odour stimulates our sense of smell. It is also interesting to note that, during pregnancy, scents that a woman previously found attractive can become distasteful to her.

Odours play an important role in the way we feel and the things we remember. If a previously unfamiliar scent is associated with a particular emotion, the next time that you smell it your mood will change accordingly. This is why lovers often have a special fragrance and send each other letters perfumed with 'their' scent. Not only is it a caring and loving thought, but the perfume reminds them of those special moments together.

Fragrance plays an important role in our lives. However, it must be remembered that it does not just evoke good memories; a particular scent can also remind us of a tragedy or unpleasant experience. However, if someone is feeling depressed, the right perfume can work wonders. A short, caring message on note paper that has had a drop or two of bergamot oil sprinkled on it, sent to a friend who is having a difficult time will immediately lift their spirits.

Perfume is a statement of our individuality — just like the clothes we wear.

## What is Perfume?

Technically, perfume is a particular combination of natural essential oils and fragrant compounds, mixed together to make a pleasing blend. To the layperson, it is simply a sweet-smelling, acceptable scent.

Perfumes are not only an enjoyable fragrance; their effectiveness is also dependent upon another dimension — time. They change over time and just like wine, some will improve, and some will not.

Perfumers expend an enormous amount of time on complicated blending to produce a truly unique scent. They will choose from millions of fragrant substances with the objective of blending the top, middle and base notes together in perfect harmony, just like a musical symphony. When modern perfumers talk of these 'notes', they are really referring to a theoretical model which is used to help describe perfume. Top notes are fresh and mouth-watering, like the citrus oils. Middle notes are warmer and more gentle to the nose, and they are derived from floral fragrances. Base notes have a woody scent, such as sandalwood and cedarwood. The musical analogy does not end here: these different notes are put together to create pleasing and delightful harmonies, which are just as challenging to their creators as the symphonies composed by Mendelssohn and Beethoven must have been.

## Choosing a Scent

Just how do you find the perfume that is right for you? It can be quite difficult to find a scent that harmonises with your body chemistry and which also suits the climate in which you live. For instance, a fragrance which appeals to your own sense of smell can be overpowering or even offensive to others.

When choosing a perfume, consider what mood you wish to portray: shy, sexy, romantic, alluring, elusive or glamorous? Keep a different scent for each occasion. You also need to bear in mind the climate and season. In cooler weather a scent tends to be more noticeable. Hot, humid conditions intensify a fragrance, and in extremely hot and dry climates a perfume almost disappears.

It is also important to take into account the way your skin reacts according to changes in diet and lifestyle, which in turn affect the way a perfume smells.

Choosing the right fragrance for you can, therefore, be a somewhat complicated business. It is not as simple as just picking up a bottle, sniffing the contents and dabbing it on. Always try a small amount first on the inside of your wrist.

## Blending Your Own Fragrance

Blending your own fragrance can be a lot of fun and a real 'learning experience'. It will help you to understand the art of perfumery and to appreciate the delicate balance between different aromatic substances.

Nearly all perfumes have top, middle, and base notes. Combining these different notes can be compared to building a house. The base notes are the foundations, the middle notes the walls and the top notes the roof. In addition to this 'main construction' there are also scents known as modifiers. These add that special touch that makes your fragrant 'house' different from the others.

It is the harmonious blending of the different notes that makes a good perfume. Top notes evaporate very quickly, middle notes not quite as fast, and base notes slowly. When making a perfume, it is important to first establish your base note, or combination of base notes, followed by your middle and top notes.

Experimenting with different fragrances is the best way to start. Remember, when you start creating these aromatic masterpieces, be sure to write down the recipes. Who knows, you may just create another Chanel No. 5!

## The Fragrant Notes

| OIL | BLENDS WELL WITH |
|---|---|

*BASE NOTES ('FOUNDATIONS')*

| | |
|---|---|
| CEDARWOOD | *Hyacinth, neroli, violet, bergamot, jasmine, rosemary and juniper.* |
| CINNAMON | *Frankincense and citrus oils.* |
| FRANKINCENSE | *All fragrances.* |
| HELIOTROPE | *Neroli, violet and stephanotis.* |
| JASMINE | *All fragrances.* |
| MUSK | *Rose, violet, jasmine, tuberose and stephanotis.* |
| MYRRH | *Lavender and spice oils.* |
| OAKMOSS | *Rose, jasmine and hyacinth.* |
| ORRISROOT | *Daphne, neroli, frangipani and rose.* |
| PATCHOULI | *Rose, bergamot, geranium, lavender, myrrh and neroli.* |
| SANDALWOOD | *Honeysuckle, daphne, violet, jasmine, neroli, frankincense and ylang-ylang.* |
| YLANG-YLANG | *Most fragrances.* |

*MIDDLE NOTES ('WALLS')*

| | |
|---|---|
| CARNATION | *Orrisroot, musk and heliotrope.* |
| DAPHNE | *Sandalwood, orrisroot and heliotrope.* |
| FRANGIPANI | *Sandalwood, heliotrope and oakmoss.* |
| GARDENIA | *Musk, sandalwood and heliotrope.* |
| GERANIUM | *All fragrances.* |
| HONEYSUCKLE | *Musk, sandalwood and heliotrope.* |
| HYACINTH | *Orrisroot and sandalwood.* |
| JASMINE | *Sandalwood, oakmoss, and most other fragrances.* |
| JONQUIL | *Orrisroot, musk and sandalwood.* |
| LAVENDER | *Most fragrances, particularly oakmoss, orrisroot, musk and sandalwood.* |
| MELISSA | *Geranium, neroli and ylang-ylang.* |

| | |
|---|---|
| ROSE | *Musk, orrisroot, oak-moss, patchouli, and most other fragrances.* |
| STEPHANOTIS | *Musk, heliotrope and sandalwood.* |
| TUBEROSE | *Musk, sandalwood and orrisroot.* |
| VIOLET | *Cedarwood, heliotrope and orrisroot.* |

*TOP NOTES ('ROOF')*

| | |
|---|---|
| BASIL | *Bergamot, geranium, neroli, melissa and lavender.* |
| BERGAMOT | *Most floral fragrances.* |
| EUCALYPTUS | *Lavender, lemon, lemon verbena, melissa and rose (gives fresh medicinal top notes).* |
| LAVENDER | *Most fragrances (gives clear herbal top notes).* |
| LEMON | *Eucalyptus, frankincense and most floral fragrances.* |
| LEMON VERBENA | *Most floral fragrances.* |
| LIME | *Most floral fragrances.* |
| NEROLI | *Most fragrances.* |
| NIAOULI | *Lavender and mints.* |
| PEPPERMINT | *Melissa and spice fragrances (gives fresh medicinal top notes).* |
| ROSEMARY | *Basil, cedarwood, frankincense, lavender, lemon and peppermint (gives clear herbal top notes).* |

The fragrances listed here are by no means exhaustive. Their purpose is to serve as a guide, and to give you a point from which to begin your experiments.

First decide what floral notes (middle notes) you would like to use. Then choose your complementary base note(s). Thirdly, add the floral notes to the selected base note (not the other way around). Finish off with a complementary top note.

As a general guide, use twice as much of the top notes to the middle notes, and again to the base notes — a ratio of 4 parts top, 2 parts middle and 1 part base would be a good formula with which to start. You will soon become very skilled in blending the different fragrances.

If the fragrance is too fresh, add a little more of the base note(s). Too heavy, add a little more of the middle or top note(s). Go slowly and sparingly and always use very small amounts. A dropper which is especially suited for essential oils will make the task that much easier.

Remember, a well constructed perfume will smell as if it is one fragrance, not a combination of elements.

## *Modifiers*

Modifiers give a special and interesting 'twist' to your fragrance, but they must be used very sparingly. It is better to use too little than to use too much.

When adding a modifier to your perfume blend, let your nose be your guide. If you can actually smell it in the blend, you have used too much. Put in more of the floral fragrance(s) to correct the problem.

Choose from any of the following fragrances to suit your particular blend:

| FRAGRANCE | OIL NOTES | BLENDS WELL WITH |
|---|---|---|
| ALLSPICE | Spicy | Daphne, bergamot and orange. |
| APPLE | Fruity | Jasmine, violet and gardenia. |
| AMOISE (MUGWORT) | Herbal | Violet and lavender. |
| BAY RUM | Spicy | Carnation, rose and violet. |
| CINNAMON | Spicy | Carnation, rose and violet. |
| CLOVE | Spicy | Carnation, rose and violet. |
| GALBANUM | Green | Jasmine, amoise (mugwort), jonquil and daphne. |
| GERANIUM | Oriental | Rose, violet, neroli and tuberose. |
| PATCHOULI | Woody | Rose, jasmine and carnation. |
| STRAWBERRY | Fruity | Jasmine, violet and gardenia. |
| THYME | Herbal | Amoise (mugwort) and lavender. |

## *A Word of Advice*

A few basic rules will help to prevent your first steps in perfume–making ending in disaster.

❋ *First decide the strength of the perfume you are going to make. 'Eau de' type perfumes are lighter than perfumes and floral waters. Put the latter in air spray atomisers, and use around the home.*

❋ *Do not try too many different scents at once — you will only confuse your nose. Introduce additional scents as your expertise increases.*

❋ *Choose scents that match your personality, moods and lifestyle. Light, refreshing perfumes are often best in the morning, for instance, while heavier, more exotic scents are usually suitable only for evening.*

❋ *Perfumes deteriorate when they are exposed to heat, light, air and moisture. Store them in dark or frosted glass bottles with airtight caps.*

# Air Sprays and Fresheners

Essential oils and other fragrant substances can be sprayed around the room, added to cleaning products, polishes and detergents, included in the household wash, blended with potpourri or burnt in a simmering pot to scent a room (see page 118).

Just a few drops of essential oil in the vacuum cleaner bag will leave behind a delightful fragrance as you clean. Placing a drop or two on a face washer and adding it to the final washing cycle will leave your clothes fragrant and fresh-smelling. It is so easy and simple to add fragrance to your world.

## AIR FRESHENER SPRAY

You might like to experiment with making your own 'personalised' combination, or use the *Air Purification Spray* or *Room Freshener* recipes given in Chapter 1, (see page 22). The following 'bacteria buster' is the air spray most commonly used in my home; it freshens every room and also kills airborne bacteria and viruses. The special blend of oils produces a delightful aroma, releasing an immediate burst which teases the senses, followed by a lingering, elusive scent which keeps rooms smelling fragrant and fresh.

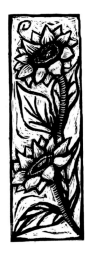

*1.5 ml bergamot essential oil*
*1 ml nutmeg essential oil*
*0.4 ml chamomile essential oil*
*0.4 ml jasmine essential oil*
*0.2 ml lavender essential oil*
*0.2 ml ylang-ylang essential oil*
*2 teaspoons methylated spirits*
*500 ml (16 fl oz) distilled water*

Dissolve all the oils in the methylated spirits. Pour into a pump-spray bottle with the distilled water. Shake mixture well. Use on a fine mist setting several times during the day and evening.

# Perfumes

Whatever the mood or occasion, scent plays an important role in our lives and has a lot to do with an individual's search for their identity. Perfume can be worn anywhere on the body but, for maximum effect, it should be applied to the various pulse points. These are found on the inside of the wrist, the crook of the elbow, at the nape of the neck, the temples, behind the knees and under the breasts.

Creating your own perfume from scratch can only be judged a success if you, and the people around you, like it. Start with a simple eau de cologne, or any of the following special blends.

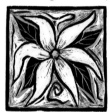
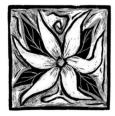

## EAU DE COLOGNE
*1.5 ml bergamot essential oil*
*1.5 ml lemon essential oil*
*35 drops orange essential oil*
*10 drops neroli essential oil*
*5 drops rosemary essential oil*
*100 ml (3½ fl oz) orrisroot perfume base (or vodka)*

Mix all ingredients and allow to stand for 48 hours. Drip through filter paper, and store in a tightly sealed bottle.

If you would like a strong scent, allow the liquid to stand for a further 4 to 6 weeks before filtering. Alternatively, the scent can be diluted by adding up to 50 per cent distilled water to the mixture.

## ROSEWATER PERFUME
*750 ml (24 fl oz) orrisroot perfume base (or vodka)*
*250 ml (8 fl oz) rosewater*
*6 ml (⅕ fl oz) rose essential oil*
*25 drops bergamot essential oil*

Mix all ingredients thoroughly and allow to stand for 10 days. Drip through filter paper into glass bottles and seal tightly.

## HUNGARY WATER
*2.5 ml (¹⁄₁₂ fl oz) rosemary essential oil*
*2.5 ml (¹⁄₁₂ fl oz) lavender essential oil*
*750 ml (24 fl oz) orrisroot perfume base (or vodka)*
*250 ml (8 fl oz) orange flower water*

Dissolve the essential oils in the alcohol. Mix with the orange flower water, and store in an airtight bottle.

## LAVENDER WATER

*570 ml (19 fl oz) orrisroot perfume base (or vodka)*
*130 ml (4½ fl oz) rosewater or distilled water*
*6 ml (⅕ fl oz) lavender essential oil*
*30 drops bergamot essential oil*

Mix all ingredients and allow to stand for 10 days. Drip through filter paper and store in a tightly sealed glass bottle.

# Floral Waters and Body Colognes

These invigorating water-based lotions can be splashed on or misted over the body with an atomiser. Depending upon the essential oils used, floral waters and body colognes can have a stimulating, toning or relaxing effect. They are ideal for use on hot summer days or nights, giving your spirits a lift by making you feel fresh and cool. They will not leave an oily residue on the skin.

These scents are also simple to make, fun to use and make an ideal gift for a friend.

## ROSE TOILET WATER

This toilet water is simple to make, and may be based on either fresh or dried rose petals.

*rose petals, sufficient*
*1 litre (35 fl oz) distilled water*
*40 ml (1½ fl oz) vodka*
*6 drops rose essential oil*

Fill a warmed, heat-resistant jar with the rose petals. Bring distilled water to the boil in an enamel or stainless steel saucepan, and add enough boiling water to cover the petals. Seal the jar and leave to cool slightly. Add the vodka to the mixture, seal again and leave until completely cool.

Strain through muslin cloth, squeezing all liquid from the petals. Add the essential oil, mix well, and store in an airtight bottle for 48 hours. Drip through filter paper and store in an airtight bottle.

## LEMON FRESH TOILET WATER
*1 generous handful lemon verbena leaves*
*1 generous handful lime scented geranium (Pelargonium nervosum) leaves*
*300 ml (10 fl oz) orrisroot perfume base (or high proof vodka)*
*2.25 ml (1/12 fl oz) lemon essential oil*
*1 ml lime essential oil*
*150 ml (5 fl oz) distilled water*

Put the herbs in a wide-mouthed glass jar, add the alcohol and seal tightly. Shake vigorously, then leave in a warm place for 14 days. Shake the contents every day. Strain through muslin, add the essential oils and distilled water and allow to stand in an airtight bottle for a further 48 hours. Drip through filter paper and store in a tightly sealed bottle.

## ELDER FLOWER SKIN REFRESHER
Splash or spray this blend over your skin when the weather is hot and humid. It is particularly delightful to use after spending a day at the beach, as it will soothe hot and sticky skin.

*2 cups (310 g/10 oz) fresh elder flowers*
*300 ml (16 fl oz) boiling water*
*150 ml (5 fl oz) vodka*
*6 drops bergamot essential oil*
*2 drops lemon essential oil*

Put the elder flowers in a ceramic bowl and add the boiling water. Cover, steep overnight, and blend with the vodka and essential oils. Allow to stand for one week in a tightly sealed bottle, then drip through filter paper.

## FRUITY BODY SPLASH
*2 tablespoons orange peel, thinly-pared*
*150 ml (5 fl oz) orrisroot perfume base (or high proof vodka)*
*10 drops orange essential oil*
*10 drops bergamot essential oil*
*5 drops lemon essential oil*
*5 drops grapefruit essential oil*
*500 ml (16 fl oz) distilled water*

Mix the orange peel with the alcohol in an airtight jar and leave to steep for 7 days. Strain, add the essential oils and distilled water, reseal and allow to stand for a further 14 days. Drip through filter paper into glass bottles and seal.

## FLORAL SKIN FRESHENER

Apply generously on hot summer days to refresh your skin and lift your spirits.

*2 cups (310 g/10 oz) fresh rose petals*
*1 cup (155 g/5 oz) fresh violet petals*
*375 ml (12 fl oz) vodka*
*14 drops rose essential oil*
*14 drops bergamot essential oil*
*750 ml (24 fl oz) distilled water*

Put the flower petals in a wide-mouthed glass jar, add the vodka and seal tightly. Leave in a warm place for 1 week. Strain, squeezing all liquid from the petals, and re-bottle. Add the essential oils and distilled water, seal and allow to stand for another week. Drip through filter paper and store in tightly sealed glass bottles.

# Colognes for the Bath or Face

Plants with sharp, fresh scents, such as mint, pine needles, fennel leaves and juniper berries, may be steeped in alcohol (such as a high proof vodka or orrisroot perfume base) and are excellent for these types of colognes. They can also be used as aftershave skin fresheners.

## PURIFYING BATH COLOGNE

*10 drops geranium essential oil*
*5 drops lemon essential oil*
*5 drops juniper essential oil*
*3 drops peppermint essential oil*
*10 ml (⅓ fl oz) vodka*
*100 ml (3½ fl oz) cider vinegar*
*600 ml (20 fl oz) distilled water*

Dissolve the essential oils in the vodka, mix with the vinegar and allow to stand in an airtight bottle for 6 weeks. Blend mixture with the distilled water and reseal, shaking well to mix, then allow to stand for a further 48 hours. Drip through filter paper and store in tightly sealed bottles with non-metallic lids.

Add a tablespoon (or more if the scent needs strengthening) to the bath after the hot water has settled.

## AFTERSHAVE SPLASH

This is a refreshing, mildly antiseptic and delightfully aromatic aftershave lotion. It is an ideal gift for men.

*10 drops rosemary essential oil*
*6 drops bay essential oil*
*6 drops lemon essential oil*
*3 drops lime essential oil*
*2 drops sage essential oil*
*10 ml (⅓ fl oz) tincture of benzoin (friar's balsam)*
*15 ml (½ fl oz) witch hazel (from the chemist)*
*50 ml (2 fl oz) rosewater*
*50 ml (2 fl oz) cider vinegar*

Dissolve the essential oils in the tincture of benzoin, and then mix with the witch hazel, ensuring that the mixture is well blended. Mix the rosewater and cider vinegar together, and then thoroughly blend the two solutions together. Store in a glass bottle with a tight-fitting, non-metallic lid.

# *Making Fragrances Linger*

Here are several suggestions as to how you can make your natural fragrances last longer.

✳ *Always apply to pulse points.*

✳ *Apply to several points, not just one.*

✳ *Don't skimp. Be generous and apply liberally so that the initial 'lift' of your fragrance is a little more intense than you actually want it to be.*

✳ *Avoid neutralising your fragrance by using unscented grooming products. Add a few drops of the same scent to your body talc and body lotion, too.*

✳ *Scent applied to the inside of your wrists tends to be removed when you wash your hands.*

# CHAPTER FOUR

# The Magic Touch

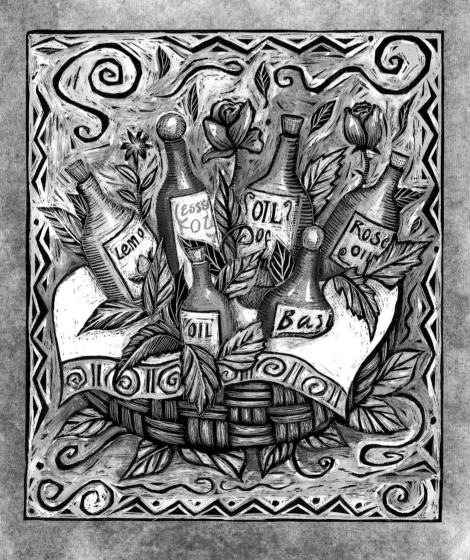

# *Massage for Health*

Massage is important in many of the body's healing processes. It can also be used as a pleasurable part of foreplay to a romantic interlude. The benefits of massage are many and greatly contribute to our overall wellbeing.

In the simplest terms, massage can be described as the art of touching. Although many underestimate its full potential — seeing it only as a pleasurable experience — massage is invaluable for enhancing human health and vitality.

When receiving a massage, the first benefit you will notice is the fragrance of the aromatics teasing your olfactory nerves. Depending on the oils selected and the needs of the individual, this fragrance can either stimulate or relax the mind and spirit.

Aromatherapy is a very powerful tool for health. The combination of touch and fragrance can relieve stress and tension, alleviate fatigue and promote deep relaxation, as well as encourage the body's organs and systems to function at optimum levels. In a world filled with anxiety, massage is one obvious solution which can help to comfort and console. It can quickly transport you from the rigours and problems of work and daily life, allowing you to feel refreshed and even euphoric.

In certain combinations, selected oils have antibacterial effects and can help to heal or relieve internal conditions and skin problems. For instance, they can improve blood circulation, speed up the elimination of old skin cells and help to improve new cell growth. Other oils, combined with the massage procedure, can help to accelerate the elimination of wastes through the body's lymph system.

More than 2000 years ago, the ancient Greeks were well aware of the benefits of massage for their athletes. It became part of their regular regime to improve their bodies' endurance and to diminish fatigue. It is also worth noting that, at the conclusion of any form of exercise, muscle recovery rate after a 5 minute rest is usually around 20%. If, however, the body is massaged in preference to just resting, the muscle recovery rate escalates to 75% or more.

When you discover aromatherapy you discover a natural and effective means of enhancing your wellbeing. Both your body and mind become vital, healthy and in tune with each other.

# Selecting Massage Oils

Choose your oils from those described in Chapter Two (see pages 40–43), or from the *Therapeutic Index* below, for the condition you wish to treat. In some instances one oil will be sufficient; in other circumstances two, three or, occasionally, four oils are combined.

You may also wish to consider the note of a particular oil, and so affect a person's mood, in addition to the other benefits obtained from the massage. To do this, refer to the guide under *Blending Your Own Fragrance* in Chapter Three (see page 47). This will also serve as a useful guide to blending oils when more than one is required for a particular massage.

## Therapeutic Index

Here you will find more than one essential oil listed for each condition. The oil listed at the beginning of each group is the one considered most appropriate for the treatment. These oil blends are to be used in massage only, and are not to be taken internally.

| CONDITION | ESSENTIAL OIL |
|---|---|
| ACNE | *Cajuput, juniper, chamomile, eucalyptus, lavender, lemongrass and sandalwood.* |
| ANXIETY | *Jasmine, lavender, marjoram, neroli, basil, bergamot, chamomile, frankincense, geranium, juniper, rose, melissa and sandalwood.* |
| APATHY | *Jasmine and rosemary.* |
| APPETITE, LOSS OF | *Chamomile, bergamot, black pepper, ginger, hyssop, myrrh and sage.* |
| ARTHRITIS | *Chamomile, cypress, sage, juniper, lemon and thyme.* |
| ATHLETE'S FOOT | *Myrrh and lavender.* |
| BRUISES | *Hyssop, calendula and fennel.* |
| BURNS AND SCALDS | *(Note: always seek medical advice for severe burns and scalds) Lavender, chamomile, eucalyptus and geranium.* |
| CAPILLARIES, BROKEN | *Chamomile, cypress, rose, lavender and neroli.* |
| CELLULITE | *Cypress, fennel and oregano.* |
| CHILBLAINS | *Lavender, lemon and camphor.* |
| CIRCULATION, POOR | *Black pepper, juniper, cypress and lavender.* |
| COLDS | *Lemon, pine and tea tree.* |

| | |
|---|---|
| COUGHS | *Cypress, eucalyptus and thyme.* |
| CRAMP | *Basil, cypress and marjoram.* |
| DANDRUFF | *Chamomile, juniper, lavender and rosemary.* |
| DEPRESSION | *Camphor, chamomile, jasmine, thyme, basil, bergamot and geranium.* |
| ECZEMA, DRY | *Chamomile, geranium, hyssop and lavender.* |
| ECZEMA, WEEPING | *Bergamot and juniper.* |
| FEVERS | *Basil, black pepper, chamomile, eucalyptus, melissa and peppermint.* |
| FLU | *Black pepper, eucalyptus, peppermint, rosemary and cypress.* |
| HAIR LOSS | *Lavender, rosemary and sage.* |
| HAY FEVER | *Chamomile, cypress, lavender, lemon, pine and rose.* |
| HEADACHE | *Chamomile, lavender, lemon and marjoram.* |
| INSECT BITES | *Lavender, basil, cinnamon, lemon, melissa, sage and thyme.* |
| INSOMNIA | *Basil, chamomile, lavender, marjoram, neroli, rose and ylang-ylang.* |
| ITCHY SKIN | *Chamomile.* |
| MENSTRUATION, PAINFUL | *Cypress, oregano, peppermint and sage.* |
| MENTAL FATIGUE | *Rosemary, basil and peppermint.* |
| MOSQUITO REPELLENT | *Eucalyptus, clove, geranium, lavender and peppermint.* |
| MUSCULAR ACHES | *Eucalyptus, lavender, rosemary and black pepper.* |
| MUSCLE STIFFNESS | *Rosemary and thyme.* |
| NAUSEA | *Peppermint, basil, black pepper, lavender and rose.* |
| NERVOUSNESS | *Basil, bergamot, chamomile, geranium, neroli and rose.* |
| NEURALGIA, FACIAL | *Chamomile, geranium, eucalyptus and peppermint.* |
| PSORIASIS | *Bergamot, cajuput and lavender.* |
| RHEUMATISM | *Rosemary, ginger, oregano, pine and thyme.* |
| SHINGLES | *Eucalyptus, geranium and peppermint.* |
| SHOCK | *Camphor, melissa, neroli and peppermint.* |
| SINUSITIS | *Basil, eucalyptus, lavender, lemon, pine and thyme.* |
| SKIN, CHAPPED | *Benzoin, patchouli, chamomile, geranium and rose.* |
| SKIN, SPOTS | *Juniper, lavender and lemon.* |
| SPRAINS | *Eucalyptus and lavender.* |
| STRESS | *Neroli and juniper.* |

# *Therapeutic Blends*

The following formulae will give you a quick guide for treating common problems with massage. Some blends can also be used to treat the problem in an inhalation, and are described accordingly.

| PROBLEM | MASSAGE OIL BLEND |
|---|---|
| ARTHRITIS | *10 drops each of juniper and lemon, 5 drops of thyme* |
| BRONCHITIS | *10 drops each of eucalyptus and niaouli, 5 drops each of hyssop and sandalwood* |
| | *Inhalation: 4 drops each of eucalyptus and niaouli, 2 drops of hyssop* |
| CELLULITE | *6 drops of eucalyptus, 8 drops each of oregano, fennel and rosemary (blend these in a hazelnut carrier oil)* |
| CIRCULATION, POOR | *12 drops each of black pepper and juniper, 8 drops of cypress* |
| COLDS AND FLU | *7 drops each of cinnamon, eucalyptus, tea tree and pine* |
| | *Inhalation (head cold): 3 drops each of basil, eucalyptus and ginger* |
| | *Inhalation (cough & cold): 3 drops each of benzoin and eucalyptus, 2 drops each of cypress and pine* |
| ECZEMA, DRY | *10 drops of calendula, 5 drops each of chamomile, geranium and lavender* |
| ECZEMA, WEEPING | *10 drops each of calendula and bergamot, 5 drops juniper* |
| MENSTRUAL PAIN | *4 drops of jasmine, 7 drops each of chamomile, clary sage and cypress* |
| MUSCULAR ACHES | *6 drops of eucalyptus, 8 drops each of bergamot, coriander and rosemary (use hazelnut oil as the carrier)* |
| MUSCULAR CRAMP | *10 drops of basil, 8 drops each of cypress and rosemary* |
| SINUS | *7 drops each of basil, eucalyptus, lavender and peppermint* |
| | *Inhalation: 2 drops each of basil, eucalyptus, lavender and peppermint* |
| STRETCH MARKS | *15 drops of lavender, 10 drops of frankincense, 5 drops of neroli* |

You will see that hazelnut oil has been recommended as the carrier oil for treating cellulite and muscular aches. Although other oils are acceptable, hazelnut penetrates the most easily and deeply, stimulating the circulation at the same time. (See *Carrier Oils* [page 63]).

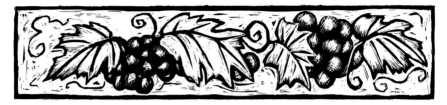

# Blending Oils for Massage

Essential oils are usually sold in glass bottles measured in millilitres (fluid ounces). Unless you buy your oils in bulk (which is far more economical), the average-sized bottle contains between 15 and 20 ml (½ and ⅔ fl oz).

Most recipes in this book express the quantity of oil to be used in drops. One millilitre equals about 20 drops of essential oil so, used carefully and correctly, your wardrobe of oils will last you a considerable time. Naturally, this will depend upon your daily usage patterns, the strength of the blend and other individual needs. Trial and error will teach you to assess these needs and recognise that some health problems, and individuals, respond to diluted blends while others require greater strength.

When you are preparing a massage oil for the first time, start with an average or middle-of-the-road strength: 10 drops of essential oil to 20 ml (⅔ fl oz) of carrier oil. Lower concentrations of essential oil usually give the best results for emotional problems, whereas higher concentrations are more suitable for physical problems.

One full body massage uses between 10 and 20 ml (⅓ and ⅔ fl oz) of carrier oil. This quantity of oil, plus the appropriate essential oils, can be adjusted proportionately, depending on the extent of the massage. When measuring oils, use an eggcup or medicine glass, and a glass dropper for accuracy.

You can premix your massage oils and store them, bearing in mind the keeping period discussed in Chapter Two (see page 36). This should only be done in circumstances where you will be using a particular blend frequently. Add 40 ml (1½ fl oz) of your chosen carrier oil, 5 ml (⅙ fl oz) avocado oil for greater penetration, 5 ml (⅙ fl oz) wheat germ oil to extend the keeping qualities, and no less than 15 drops and no more than 30 drops of your chosen essential oils to an amber-coloured glass. Do not forget to date and label the bottle.

# *Carrier Oils*

A carrier oil is just that — it carries the beneficial essential oils which, in concentrated form, may irritate the skin. It also acts as a lubricant, allowing the hands to glide smoothly over the skin.

The most suitable carrier oils are cold-pressed vegetable oils. A carrier oil should have little or no smell, be 100% pure, and should also be beneficial to the skin. Those most suitable are:

ALMOND OIL — *This is by far the most popular of the carrier oils. It has little smell, is rich in protein and is both an emollient and nourishing skin moisturiser. It is also very slow to become rancid, and is therefore an excellent choice when making up blends which are to be bottled and stored.*

APRICOT KERNEL OIL — *This has the same properties as almond oil, but it is far more expensive.*

GRAPESEED OIL — *A very fine and clear oil; it does not make skin greasy to touch but gives it a satin smooth finish.*

HAZELNUT OIL — *This penetrates quicker, deeper and more easily than all the other vegetable oils. It nourishes the skin and stimulates the circulation, making it ideal for muscular problems.*

JOJOBA OIL — *Pronounced ho-ho-ba, this is a good 'keeping' oil meaning it is slow to go rancid. It can be used to treat acne and, in general body massages, will make skin feel smooth and satiny.*

OLIVE OIL — *This oil is both warming and calming, making it good for rheumatism and to help relieve the itching caused by some skin disorders. However, its own natural scent can overpower the fragrance of any essential oils that are blended with it.*

SESAME OIL — *This oil keeps extremely well. It can be used for treating skin disorders such as eczema and psoriasis.*

SOYA OIL — *This oil has a nice 'feel' for massage work. It does not become sticky under pressure.*

SUNFLOWER OIL — *Although this oil has limited keeping qualities, its advantage lies in the fact that it contains vitamin F. Vitamin F is that group containing the unsaturated fatty acids. It controls the metabolic rate, takes care of the cholesterol balance, and prevents eczema and dull, dry hair. It also plays a role in the correction of dandruff and acne, and regulates over-activity of the sebaceous glands. This vitamin is vital to the continuing health of the cell membranes.*

# Add-in Oils

There are a number of other oils, apart from the essential oils, which can also be included in small quantities to help form the base. These 'add-in' oils exert special properties, such as increasing penetrative and keeping qualities. They are:

| | |
|---|---|
| AVOCADO OIL | *Both nourishing and penetrating; useful for fatty areas and for inclusion in muscle preparations.* |
| CALENDULA OIL | *Exerts a beneficial effect in healing chapped and cracked skin.* |
| CARROT OIL | *This oil is rich in many vitamins, and will tone and rejuvenate the skin. An excellent choice for neck massages.* |
| EVENING PRIMROSE OIL | *Use this oil when scaly skin and/or dandruff is evident.* |
| WHEAT GERM OIL | *This is a natural preservative (anti-oxidant) and will extend the keeping time of massage blends. This oil is also nourishing and rich in vitamin E.* |

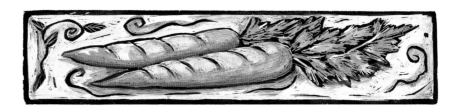

# When to Avoid Massage

Although in most circumstances the use of aromatherapy is highly beneficial to the body's natural healing process, there are certain times when it should be avoided.

✳ *After a very hot bath, sauna or steam bath. For at least an hour afterwards, the skin will be eliminating excess heat, toxins and surplus moisture.*

✳ *Areas that may cause discomfort. This also includes areas where there are fractures, broken skin, varicose veins, torn muscles and ligaments, sprains, bruises, swellings and rashes.*

✳ *When a person has a temperature, fever or viral disease. The latter situation is particularly important, as massage may cause the infection to spread further via the lymphatic system.*

✳ *When someone is recovering from a recent serious operation.*

✳ *If the person to be massaged has heart trouble or acute back pain.*

*✳ Never give a massage straight after a meal, especially in the abdominal area.*

*✳ If you have any doubts at all about a person's health, do not give them a massage.*

# Putting on the Pressure

Sensual massage with a friend provides an enjoyable interlude and requires little, if any, pressure in its application. With a therapeutic massage, pressure applied to specific points during the treatment can help to restore a balanced energy flow.

Reflexology, a more specific form of pressure point massage, deals specifically with hands and feet. It is not my intention to cover this subject in detail — it would be a book in itself! — but I would like to point out the use of reflexology as an antidote to some everyday problems.

Most of us feel tired and exhausted after a hectic day. A hand and foot massage is a marvellous way of reviving the body without having to undertake a full body massage. Not only is it something you can easily do yourself, but it can also be used to alleviate particular problems.

## QUICK FOOT MASSAGE

Before commencing the massage, pour the oil into your hands and hold the left foot firmly. Press along the underneath area and upper surface for about 20 seconds. This will induce a marvellous feeling of relaxation.

Next, place your left foot over your knee. Press, rub and pull each toe, and knead the sole with your knuckles. Then place the fingers of both hands on the sole and the thumbs, pointing toward the toes, on top of the foot; stroke down from the ankles to the toes. Repeat the procedure with your other foot.

## HAND MASSAGE

The pressure points on your hands are easily located, and may be worked for half a minute at a time. They can be found on the pads of each finger and the thumb, in the centre of the palm (this is known as the solar plexus point), and also slightly up and to the left (or right) of this point, between the thumb and little finger. To massage, cradle your hand and support it with the fingers of your other hand, then apply pressure by alternately bending and straightening your thumb.

### HEADACHES, STRESS AND NECK PAIN

Massage the pad of each thumb, from the knuckle joint to the tip, and concentrate on that area closest to the forefinger.

### FATIGUE

Counteract fatigue by stimulating the adrenal glands. Treat both hands by applying pressure to that point slightly up and to the left (or right) of the solar plexus point.

### INSOMNIA

If you have trouble unwinding or can not sleep because of tension or racing thoughts, work the solar plexus point of both hands. Work each hand for at least 1 minute.

### HEAD COLD

Congested sinuses, and the dull aching headache associated with them, can be relieved by working the reflex points (or pads) at the end of each finger.

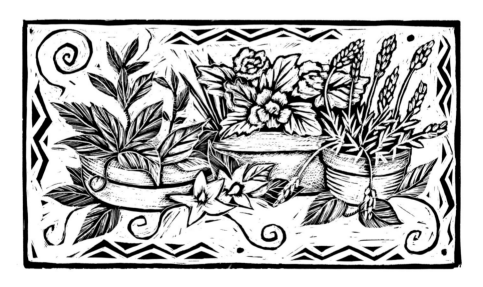

# The Art of Touching

We human beings subconsciously rely on our tactile sense, to an enormous extent, to keep us in touch with the reality of life. It is an almost automatic reaction to want to reach out and touch an object or painting you consider beautiful. When we meet, we shake hands, kiss, hug, cuddle or touch — all of which reassure us. Physical contact is essential in order for us to feel accepted, loved and secure. Similarly, when we massage one another we are conveying reassurance and understanding through the simple art of touching.

Through massage, an individual can be comforted and consoled, while at the same time their stress and accumulated tension are alleviated. At some time most of us will struggle with our emotions: they can cause depression, anxiety, irritability and downright nastiness. Yet we often remain oblivious to the disturbing physical effects of this negativity. Muscles become tense, necks stiffen, headaches persist, bodies ache all over with a general feeling of lethargy, which are all symptoms of stress that we often just put up with.

With the right blend of essential oils, aromatherapy can release inner emotional tensions, and relieve muscle stiffness and soreness.

Our circulatory system can be affected by diet, exercise and lifestyle. Massage aids the movement of blood from the head to the extremities and back again. And, unlike physical exercise, the heartbeat is not increased as a result. When the circulation is stimulated, lifeless, dull skin improves and regains a better texture and a more radiant glow. At the same time, newly-formed cells will be receiving a maximum supply of nutrients. This is an important factor in successfully treating cellulite.

A good massage on a regular basis promotes both inner and outer health. It encourages lymphatic drainage, cleanses the body of unwanted toxins and reduces discomfort and pain. Gentle strokes and pressure mimic the pumping action of the muscles, thus speeding the lymph flow through the body. Pain 'information' is prevented from reaching the brain, which makes massage especially helpful for backaches, period pain and stiff necks, and during childbirth.

## *Movements and Strokes*

Variation in movement is important for a quality massage. The different techniques described here aid in soothing tension, promoting relaxation, boosting blood and lymph circulation, improving muscle tone and the flexibility of the joints, and in reviving energy levels.

The main movements are:

EFFLEURAGE • *Gliding the hands with long, even strokes over the surface of the skin. Generally a light, stimulating movement.*

TAPOTEMENT • *Short, quick blows with your hands or fingers. These movements stimulate nerves and muscles, and boost circulation. Some of the techniques are: hacking (edge of palm), slapping (flat of the hand), tapping (fingertips), cupping (cup-shaped hands), beating (edge of fist).*

PETRISSAGE • *Kneading of muscle tissue. Includes pressing, squeezing, rolling and picking up the muscles. Performed with hands and thumbs and, for small areas, with the thumb and forefinger.*

FRICTION • *Rapid, circular pressure over a particular area, using the palms or thumbs and fingertips.*

VIBRATION • *Rapid back-and-forth 'trembling' pressure movements, using either the fingers or hands.*

## *Creating the Atmosphere*

A massage cannot be truly effective if the room that it is being carried out in is ablaze with light, full of loud noise, or otherwise adversely affected by external disturbances. Massage requires a comfortable, relaxing, warm atmosphere, situated away from chilly draughts and distractions.

The room should be properly warmed in advance — about 21°C (70°F) is fine — and you should have gentle rhythmic music playing. This will help to relax the person receiving the massage and will also help the masseur to maintain flowing even strokes. A fragrant potpourri, incense burner or simmering pot will help to create a friendly and relaxed atmosphere or, depending on the fragrance chosen, a sensual and romantic setting.

If possible, it is best to carry out a massage on a table specially designed for this purpose. Otherwise, a thick foam mat covered with blankets, and topped with a sheet to catch any oil splashes, will do.

Never massage on a bed or mattress, as they are too soft for the massage strokes to be effective.

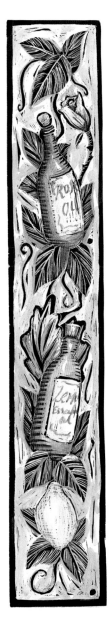

## *Tips for a More Enjoyable Massage*

In addition to creating the right atmosphere, the following tips will help to make the massage a more enjoyable experience.

✳ *Focus fully on the massage and on the person being massaged.*

✳ *Support the body part which is being massaged.*

✳ *When massaging the front of the body, place a small pillow underneath the head and another under the knees. For a back massage, remove the pillow under the head.*

✳ *Try to keep all distractions to an absolute minimum.*

✳ *Ask your partner if there are any particular tension spots that need special attention. Likewise, check if there are any spots that should be avoided, such as skin eruptions or bruises.*

✳ *Maintain a constant, even rhythm in your movements.*

✳ *Silence is the golden rule. Any discussion about what you are doing will only interfere with full sensual appreciation.*

✳ *Always remember to balance your movements.*

✳ *If you are receiving the massage, empty your mind of all thoughts. Allow your body to hang loose, to become limp and relaxed.*

✳ *To maximise the benefits of a neck and shoulder massage, have a moderately warm shower first. Do not have the water too hot or your skin will not absorb the beneficial oils.*

✳ *If you are giving the massage, concentrate on breathing regularly, and more slowly and deeply than normal. This will help you to establish a good, constant rhythm and will prevent you from tiring too quickly.*

✳ *Keep your partner warm. When you have finished massaging an area, cover it with warm towels.*

# Giving a Massage

Before starting to give a massage, ensure that your hands are clean and warm: rub them together for a few seconds if they are not, as cold hands on someone's back are not the ideal way to begin a massage!

Start with the back, and then the rest of the body in the following order: legs, feet, arms, chest and stomach, and then head, neck and shoulders.

## Back Massage

Ask the recipient to lie face down with their arms comfortably positioned along their sides or, if it is more comfortable for them, place a cushion under their forehead. Before you start, it is important to establish contact with the person being massaged. Do this by placing one of your hands on the crown of their head and the other at the base of their spine for a few seconds. While you are doing this, allow yourself to relax by breathing slowly and deeply.

Pour about a teaspoon of your selected massage oil into one hand (you can always take more later if you need it). Rub your hands together and stroke the whole of the back evenly with the oil.

Place your hands on one side of the spine, with your fingers pointing upward. Start massaging from the base of the back, working up from the buttocks and stroking lightly up the back to the base of the neck. Then slide your hands across the shoulders and bring them down lightly to your starting position. As the skin begins to warm up, you can gradually apply firmer pressure.

Continue to massage using long effleurage strokes, moving your hands to one side of the body. Start to knead the flesh, using petrissage, working up the back and across the top of the shoulders. There is very little flesh on the back, however it is still possible to knead and squeeze the shoulders, hips and buttocks. On the less fleshy areas knead more lightly, using just your thumb and forefinger. Repeat on the opposite side of the body.

Start again at the buttocks, using small friction movements along either side of the spine. Work up to the neck, over the shoulder blades and back down to the hips. Use both hands simultaneously to apply pressure to the muscles, but not to the bones.

Follow with gentle tapotement on the back and more energetic movements on the buttocks. Finish off with a few long, slow effleurage strokes; conclude by resting both hands lightly on the small of the back for a few seconds.

## *Leg Massage*

Start and finish on the back of one leg at a time. Put a little oil in the palm of your hand, gently rub your hands together and run them up the back of the first leg, pausing at the knee, then continuing upward. Stroke lightly down the leg and firmly back up to the buttocks — this encourages the flow of blood and lymph. Do this several times, being careful never to apply pressure to the backs of the knees. Knead any cellulite spots in the thighs and follow with effleurage strokes. Finish by running your hand up to the top of the thigh and sliding your hands off and outwards.

Repeat the procedure on the other leg. This time finish by running your hands up to the top of the thigh, and over the back to the shoulders. Rest your hands here for a few seconds, then slide them outwards and off. Ask the recipient to roll over. Remember to use towels to keep the person receiving the massage warm while you work on the front of their legs.

Place your hands across the first leg and begin stroking sideways, one hand after the other, from the instep to the top of the thigh then back down again. Do this several times, applying firm pressure as you go up and light, gentle strokes as you come down. Next, massage around the knee and ankle using your fingers to make small circular movements. Finish with long, gentle effleurage strokes from the ankles to the tops of the thighs.

Move to the foot, lift the leg slightly, and bring your thumbs up over the arch to the Achilles tendon, kneading in a circular motion from the sides of the heel up to the calf. Finish off by knuckle-kneading the sole and arch with the flat part of the knuckles.

Repeat the procedure with the other leg.

## *Foot Massage*

Whether enjoyed alone or as part of a complete body massage, a foot massage is a real treat. However, feet should be bathed before you start — smelly feet are offensive.

Put a small amount of oil in the palm of your hand and lightly rub your hands together. Place one under the sole of the foot and the other on top. Gently stroke both hands up to the heel and down to the big toe several times, working the oil well into the foot.

Next, place your hands on each ankle, thumbs resting on top. Commence circular kneading movements all around the ankle and foot, then knead up and down the top part of the foot with your thumbs, pressing the sole from beneath with your fingers.

Move to the toes and knead up and down each one between your thumb and forefinger. Then wrap your hands around the foot, so your thumbs meet under the sole, while your fingers rest on the top, and knead the entire sole between your thumbs and fingers. You will need to use good firm pressure, as the sole is a heavily padded spot. Rest your thumbs on the heel and slide along from the heel to the toes, moving from the sides of the foot to the centre of the sole. Repeat this movement several times, again using firm, strong strokes.

Repeat the procedure with the other foot.

## Arm Massage

Rub a little oil between your hands. Take hold of one of the recipient's hands and, with your free hand, stroke the outside of their arm from the wrist up. Do this several times, then repeat the procedure on the inside of the arm. Knead any problem areas or cellulite and finish off with long effleurage strokes up and down the arm. Repeat with the other arm.

## Massaging the Chest and Stomach

Rub a teaspoon of oil between the palms of your hands. Commence by stroking down the neck and out towards the shoulders; do this several times.

Then move from the neck area down over the collarbone to the chest, starting with light, gentle strokes, and gradually increasing the pressure. Friction massage the entire chest. With a female, however, avoid the delicate breast area unless, of course, you are very familiar with that person. Then you can use very gentle and light stroking movements across the breasts with your fingertips. This will simply add enjoyment to the massage rather than be of any therapeutic value.

Next, stroke lightly towards the stomach. With the palm of one hand, stroke firmly over the whole of the abdomen several times in a clockwise direction, then repeat the procedure with the other hand. Follow with petrissage, gently kneading and squeezing the flesh round the hips and waist. Change to effleurage and gently massage upwards from the abdomen, moving each hand up the rib cage to just beneath the armpits and then lightly gliding the hands back down. Repeat several times.

Finish by gently stroking the whole chest and stomach area, then lightly glide your fingertips up to the shoulders and gently back down again over the full length of the body.

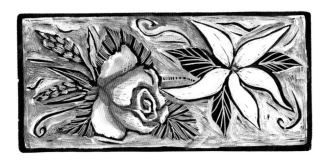

## *Head, Neck and Shoulders*

First, focus on the recipient's neck. Place your hands on one side of their neck and make small circular movements with your fingers. Massage along the sides and back of the neck, from the base of the skull to the shoulders. Repeat these movements on the other side of the neck.

Cradle the base of the recipient's skull in both your hands, letting your thumbs hang free. Stroke back and forth on the neck, pressing up against the muscles. Without changing this position, begin to massage the base of the skull with your fingers, using a vibrating motion.

Next, place one hand over the top of the recipient's head and the other at the base of their skull to support it. Press down with your top hand, moving back and forth in circles from the hairline to the back of the head. Then gently lift the head and continue down the back of the neck. Finish massaging the head by kneading the scalp with small, circular movements, using your fingers. (Do not use oil on the scalp as it is self-lubricating.) Place your fingertips over the top of the recipient's shoulders, with your thumbs sitting on the base of their neck. Begin working your fingertips and thumbs well into the muscles, using rhythmic, circular, kneading movements. Thoroughly work all tense areas on the sides of the neck.

## Facial Massage

Start by placing one hand flat across the recipient's forehead, fingers facing to the side. Stroke straight down the bridge of the nose, immediately replacing the first hand with your other hand, thus giving a smooth hand-over-hand action.

Place the fingers of both hands on the recipient's forehead, facing down toward the eyes. Commence slow, circular, gentle kneading from the middle of the forehead up and out to the temples and sides of the head.

Move to the cheeks, placing one hand on each and gently massaging with an oscillating movement. Continue down below the jaw and chin. Move to the mouth and massage the surrounding muscles firmly yet gently, by circling the lips with your index fingertips. Still using your fingertips, massage any areas of the face you have not yet reached.

Finish by pressing all around the outer ear using the pads of the first two fingers. Continue the same movement under the ear, putting a bit more pressure on the bony parts. Do this several times, then repeat on the other ear.

## Self Body Massage

Pour a teaspoon of oil into your palm and rub your hands together, then apply oil to the breasts and buttocks with a circular motion. Using a small amount of additional oil, rub your solar plexus six times in an anticlockwise direction; then stroke any residual oil upwards over your stomach with both hands.

Add another teaspoon of oil to your palm, rub your hands together, and massage each arm with firm strokes from the hand to the shoulder. Finish by deeply, yet gently, kneading up your arm with your fingers.

Using one more teaspoon of oil, work upwards over your legs with deep, firm strokes. Massage from each ankle to the top of the thigh, working with both hands.

## Self Facial Massage

Before commencing a facial massage, ensure that your face has been thoroughly cleansed of grease, grime, dirt and make-up.

First, place your hands in front of your face so that your fingers rest on your forehead and your thumbs rest just below your cheeks. Pressing gently, draw your fingers and thumbs towards your ears and away from your face. This helps to release tension from your forehead.

Pour two teaspoons of your chosen oil mix into a shallow saucer. Dip your fingers lightly into the oil and rub your hands together. Using gentle strokes, start massaging under your chin and up over your face, circling the eyes in an anticlockwise direction (as you look at your fingers).

Using a little more oil, gently massage your throat and run your fingers up over your face again. Place your fingers at the centre of your forehead and commence light, yet firm, circular movements, massaging towards the temples and off at the hairline. Repeat this two or three times, finishing by pressing hard with your fingers in the middle of your forehead for a few seconds.

Massage behind your ears using small circular movements, and then press all around the outer ear using the pads of the first two fingers.

Finish the massage by placing your thumbs on your chin, and then pulling them along the jawbone to each ear, using gentle, but firm, pressure. Do this four times.

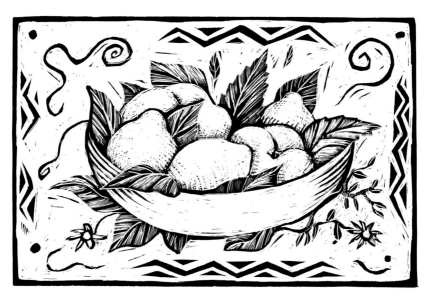

# CHAPTER FIVE

# Fragrant Beauty

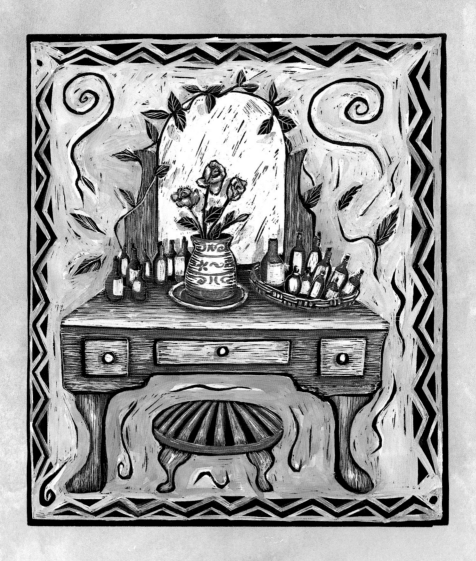

# Essential Oils and Your Skin

Although skin care preparations alone will not give your skin a healthy glow, the regular use of essential oils, either singly or in combination in creams and lotions, will keep your skin looking healthy and supple.

The skin is made up of three distinct layers: the first, or lower level, is called the subcutaneous or basal layer, followed by the dermis, and then the epidermis. The subcutaneous layer contains muscles and fatty tissue, while the sensory nerves, blood and lymph vessels, sebaceous glands and hair follicles are all located in the epidermis. Skin cells are made in the dermis and travel up to the epidermis and, in doing so, constantly renew themselves.

Essential oils will penetrate to this bottom layer of skin and so they are able to exert their beneficial effects. Certain oils can nourish the newly-formed cells, while others help to stimulate the cell renewal process with their regenerative qualities. It must be remembered, though, that these results will not be instantaneous; new skin cells can take three to four months to reach the epidermis.

Essential oils work to help slow the cosmetic effects of the ageing process. Their nourishing and regenerative properties stimulate the reproduction rate of new skin cells, reducing the time it takes for new skin to grow and for the removal of dead cells. At the same time, essential oils prevent congestion of the eliminative process of the skin and expedite the removal of toxins, improve circulation, act as bactericides and anti-inflammatories and help to calm sensitive and damaged skin. However, natural skin care products are not the sole answer, and are by no means 'miracle products'. A holistic approach, which includes regular exercise and a good diet, is also essential to keep the body trim and the skin soft and supple.

## Looking Good, Feeling Good

Your face is the most expressive part of your body. It instantly communicates your moods and personality when you meet someone, so it is very important to keep it in top condition. It is also important to have an understanding of the different skin types and, therefore, to understand which natural skin care products will give the best results. It is the activity of the sebaceous glands that determines what type of skin you have. The four main skin types are dry, oily, sensitive and normal. Most people do not have skin which falls into a single category but is, instead, a combination of dry and oily skin, with the oily areas being found along the hairline and forehead, and in a central strip down the face. If there is a large difference between skin areas, you must first identify them and then treat them separately, using different products formulated for the appropriate areas.

Normal skin is clear, supple and soft: it is neither too dry nor too oily, and it is not overly sensitive to sun, climate or environment.

Dry skin looks dull, and feels tight after washing. It needs constant protection to avoid flaking and peeling.

Sensitive, delicate skin reacts badly to sunlight or irritants by burning. It does not tan well and will quite easily develop rashes, blotches or spots on exposure to new substances.

Oily skin will feel soft and supple, but often look too shiny. It is usually prone to outbreaks of spots.

Caring for your skin with a regular routine of cleansing, toning and moisturising will not wind back the clock. It will, however, help skin to remain firm and healthy. Always remember the following tips:

❋ *Be gentle when applying preparations; do not irritate or drag the skin.*

❋ *Smooth lotions and oils on, then blot off any excess after about 15 minutes.*

❋ *Avoid extreme heat or cold as both are bad for the skin.*

❋ *Cleanse facial skin regularly.*

❋ *Do not over cleanse, or clog the pores with moisturising creams.*

❋ *Avoid harsh toning.*

# Cleansing the Face

A daily cleansing routine is the first and single most important step in good skin care. It entails removing all the grime and dirt which accumulates on your skin every day.

Natural cleansers based on essential oils in a vegetable or nut oil base, will not only gently cleanse the skin, but will nourish it at the same time. Soap, on the other hand, can disrupt the skin's acid mantle and cannot deeply cleanse the pores. All make-up is predominantly based on either wax or oil so a cleansing lotion or cream that is either an oil or an oil/wax combination is required to remove it.

When gently massaged into the skin, a natural oil cleanser frees particles of grime, dirt, grease and stale make-up, without being harsh.

The cleanser should then be wiped off with a soft piece of sterile cloth so that it does not become absorbed into the skin along with the suspended particles of grime.

Oils suitable for use as a cleansing base are: avocado or wheat germ for dry skin, almond and sunflower for oily skin, and grapeseed, sunflower and sesame for normal or sensitive skin types. Wheat germ oil can be added to all recipes, to act as a natural preservative, in amounts of no more than 10% of the total volume. Essential oils such as rosemary, chamomile, lemon, lavender or geranium are suitable additions to the base oil, and will suit all skin types.

## ALL PURPOSE CLEANSER
This is suitable for all skin types and is excellent for removing make-up.

*65 ml (2 fl oz) grapeseed oil*
*25 ml (1 fl oz) sesame oil*
*10 ml (⅓ fl oz) wheat germ oil*
*4 drops lavender essential oil*
*1 drop chamomile essential oil*

Blend all the oils together thoroughly, adding the essential oils last. Store in an airtight, amber-coloured glass bottle. Always shake well before use. To use, pour a little of the oil into the palm of one hand and warm by rubbing the palms together. Smooth over the entire face and neck, and then lightly massage into the skin using small, circular movements.

Gently wipe away all traces of the cleanser with a face flannel wrung out in tepid water, rinsing at least twice more with hot water. When all traces of oil have been removed, splash the skin with cold water and pat dry with a towel. Tone and moisturise. Warning: People with overly sensitive skin, dilated red veins or broken capillaries should exercise care so as not to aggravate any existing problem.

## LAVENDER CLEANSER
Use this to cleanse both normal and disturbed skin.

*50 ml (2 fl oz) jojoba oil*
*40 ml (1½ fl oz) almond oil*
*10 ml (⅓ fl oz) wheat germ oil*
*10 drops lavender essential oil*

Prepare and use as for the *All Purpose Cleanser* above.

## RICH CLEANSING CREAM

This is especially suitable for dry or dehydrated skin.

*10 g (⅓ oz) anhydrous lanolin*
*5 g (⅙ oz) beeswax*
*40 ml (1½ fl oz) almond oil*
*20 ml (⅔ fl oz) avocado oil*
*5 ml (⅙ fl oz) wheat germ oil*
*40 ml (1½ fl oz) distilled water*
*3 drops tincture of benzoin (friar's balsam)*
*3 drops rose essential oil*
*3 drops geranium essential oil*

Melt the lanolin and beeswax in an enamel or stainless steel double saucepan over a low heat. When completely liquefied, stir in prewarmed vegetable oils and distilled water until well blended. Remove mixture from heat, pour into a ceramic bowl, and allow to cool slightly. Add tincture of benzoin and essential oils, and stir vigorously until mixture is cool and of a creamy texture. Store in a sterilised glass jar with a tight-fitting screw top. To use, apply a small amount to facial skin and massage in gently. Then remove all traces of the cleanser with a soft piece of clean cloth.

## NECK CLEANSER

Quite often necks are forgotten when it comes to cleansing. Although any of the previous lotions and creams will work effectively, this cleansing treatment is particularly appropriate for sloughing off dead skin cells which can cause discolouration of the skin on the neck.

*2 teaspoons finely ground almonds*
*½ teaspoon jojoba oil*
*½ teaspoon almond oil*
*2 drops geranium essential oil*

Mix all the ingredients together to form a soft paste, adding the essential oil last. Apply the cleanser to the neck and chest area, massaging it in gently with upward and outward movements.

Rinse off with the following pH facial tonic water:

*2 drops lemon essential oil*
*5 ml (⅙ fl oz) witch hazel solution (from the chemist)*
*100 ml (3½ fl oz) distilled water*

Dissolve the essential oil in the witch hazel solution, then blend with the distilled water. Use this tonic to wash the neck and chest area until all traces of the cleanser have been removed. Splash with any remaining tonic or clean water, and pat dry gently with a towel.

# Facial Saunas

A facial sauna promotes perspiration, which encourages the pores of the skin to expel impurities and dirt. This leaves your face feeling clean and refreshed. The addition of essential oils to a facial sauna will increase this cleansing ability, and will often improve the texture of normal skin. Facial saunas are particularly useful for treating acne and excessive sebum (oil) discharge.

Choose essential oils which are most appropriate to your needs from any of the following:

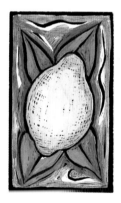

| SUITABLE FOR | ESSENTIAL OIL |
|---|---|
| CLEANSING AND SOOTHING | *Chamomile, geranium, lavender, rose and neroli.* |
| AGEING SKIN | *Frankincense, rose and neroli.* |
| NORMAL SKIN | *Lemon, lavender, chamomile and neroli.* |
| INGRAINED DIRT | *Chamomile and fennel.* |
| OILY SKIN AND EXCESSIVE SEBUM (OIL) | *Clary sage, grapefruit and juniper.* |
| ACNE | *Chamomile and lavender* |

To prepare your facial sauna, add 2 drops of essential oil to a bowl of steaming water. Hold your face over the bowl and cover your head with a towel large enough to form a tent, and so prevent the steam from escaping. Steam cleanse for no longer than 10 minutes, ensuring that you do not overexpose your skin to the heat.

Facial saunas should not be used at all on very dry skin because it is often adversely affected by heat. The steam and heat may also affect people with overly sensitive skin or dilated red veins, and those who have heart trouble, experience difficulty in breathing or suffer from asthma.

# *Face Masks*

Face masks cleanse and soothe the skin, and also help to draw out hard-to-remove grime from clogged pores, blackheads and dead skin. A face mask can be made from clay mixed with vegetable or base oils, essential oils, and vegetable or fruit juice and pulp.

Clays suitable for a face mask are:

KAOLIN (OR CHINA CLAY)   *A very fine, pure white clay powder that has an astringent effect and removes impurities while it cleanses. Use on normal to oily skins.*

FULLER'S EARTH   *A soft brown clay that can be used on troubled skin or acne, and on oily to normal-textured skin. It is very stimulating and has a cleansing action that removes dead skin cells.*

Both clays are readily available from your chemist.

## REJUVENATING MASK
This facial mask will rejuvenate, purify, tone and soothe the skin.

*4 tablespoons clay*
*vegetable or fruit juice and pulp*
*oatmeal*
*1½ tablespoons brewer's yeast*
*vegetable oil (you may include more than one)*
*apple cider vinegar, if the mask is for oily skin*
*essential oil(s)*

Mix together all the ingredients, adding sufficient oil, juices and pulp to make a thick paste. Add the essential oils last.

Apply mask to the face, avoiding the area around your eyes and lips. Leave on for about 10 minutes until the mask begins to feel tight, then gently remove with tepid water. Your skin will feel silky smooth, clean and healthy.

If the mask feels uncomfortable or begins to burn your skin, remove it immediately. Do not apply a face mask if you have any broken areas of skin.

## *Oils and Other Ingredients*

The following oils, vegetables and fruit can be used in a face mask for your particular skin type:

SENSITIVE AND DELICATE SKIN • *Alfalfa, celery and potato juice, aloe vera juice. Almond, olive and avocado oils. One teaspoon of evening primrose oil, 2 drops of carrot oil and 1 drop of chamomile essential oil.*

INGRAINED DIRT, SKIN ERUPTIONS AND ACNE • *Aloe vera juice, apple cider vinegar, cucumber, orange juice, and strawberries. Almond, avocado and wheat germ oils. One drop each of lavender and chamomile essential oils.*

OILY SKIN • *Any of the vegetable and fruits for* Acne *(see above), and apple cider vinegar. Either almond, hazelnut or grapeseed oils. One drop each of rosemary and lavender essential oils.*

NORMAL SKIN • *Aloe vera juice and carrot juice. Kelp, papaya and egg yolk. Apricot kernel, almond, avocado or wheat germ oils. One drop of geranium essential oil.*

DRY SKIN • *Any of the ingredients for* Normal Skin *(see above). Either avocado, jojoba or almond oils. Two drops of carrot oil and 1 drop of rose essential oil.*

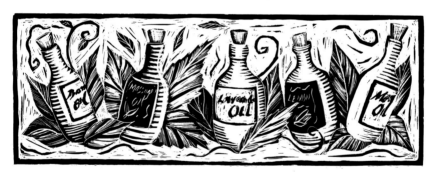

### HONEY WHEAT GERM MASK

A nourishing and cleansing mask that is especially good for removing blackheads.

*5 tablespoons honey*
*1 tablespoon wheat germ oil*
*1 drop lavender essential oil*
*1 drop lemongrass essential oil*

Combine essential oils in a glass dropper and use 1 drop.
Prepare and use as for *Rejuvenating Mask* (see page 82).

# *Tonics and Astringents*

Toning facial skin is the next important step in your daily skin care routine. Skin tonics stimulate the circulation, reduce oiliness, and help to refine the pores and the skin's texture. By redressing the skin's pH balance, toners will normalise the skin's acid mantle. Those formulated for oily skin also remove excess sebum (oil) and restrict sebum secretion.

Astringents stimulate the skin, but because of their drying effect they should only be used on skin with large open pores. They should not be applied to acne or any other type of skin blemish as they can quite easily exacerbate the problem. Instead, use a tonic especially formulated for this condition.

## *Toners*

Distilled water can be used as a base for toners for all skin types. My wife prefers to use rosewater, which is readily available from the chemist. It makes a perfect base, no matter what type of skin you have, and it is soothing and softening to the skin.

The base toner recipe is as follows:

*75 ml (2½ fl oz) rosewater*
*25 ml (1 fl oz) chamomile infusion (see recipe page 85)*
*essential oil (refer to list below for quantity)*

Put all the ingredients in a sterilised, airtight glass bottle, shake well to mix and allow to stand for 48 hours. Drip through filter paper, re-bottle and use as needed.

| TONER FOR | ESSENTIAL OILS |
|---|---|
| TIRED, SAGGING SKIN | *1 drop chamomile, 2 drops frankincense* |
| OILY SKIN | *1 drop neroli, 1 drop chamomile, 1 drop lavender* |
| DRY SKIN | *1 drop sandalwood, 1 drop neroli* |
| SENSITIVE SKIN | *Change the ratio of rosewater and chamomile infusion to 50:50, then add 1 drop each of chamomile and rose.* |
| NORMAL SKIN | *1 drop neroli, 1 drop rose* |
| SPOTS AND ACNE | *Change the base to 75 ml (2½ fl oz) lavender infusion (see recipe page 85) and 25 ml (1 fl oz) rosewater, then add 1 drop each of lavender and juniper.* |

## *Making the Infusion*

Put 3 teaspoons of dried chamomile or lavender buds, whichever is appropriate to your needs, in an enamel or stainless steel pan and cover with 1½ cups (12 fl oz) of distilled water. Bring to boiling point, reduce heat, cover and simmer for 30 minutes, adjusting the amount of distilled water if necessary. Remove from heat, cool, and strain through muslin cloth, squeezing any remaining liquid from the flowers. Add the required amount to the recipe, and prepare as directed.

## *Astringents*

Here you may use either distilled water or rosewater as the base, to which is added white wine vinegar and the appropriate essential oils.

The astringent recipe is as follows:

*essential oils*
*15 ml (½ fl oz) white wine vinegar (or apple cider vinegar for oily skin)*
*85 ml (3 fl oz) rosewater*

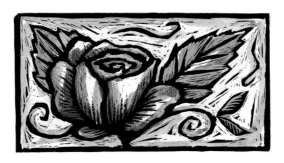

Dissolve the essential oils in the vinegar and blend with the rosewater. Cap securely with a non-metallic lid, shake well to mix and drip through filter paper.

For excessively oily skin, replace the white wine vinegar with apple cider vinegar.

| ASTRINGENT FOR | ESSENTIAL OIL |
|---|---|
| OILY SKIN | *1 drop chamomile, 1 drop neroli, 1 drop lavender* |
| MATURE SKIN | *2 drops frankincense, 1 drop neroli* |
| NORMAL SKIN | *2 drops rose, 1 drop neroli* |

# *Moisturising the Face*

Both cleansing and toning tend to dry facial skin slightly, and to remove some of the natural oils. A good moisturiser will help to replace these, keeping your skin supple and protecting it against moisture loss and external damage, dirt and grime. A natural moisturiser can counteract the effects of drying, chapping and roughening caused by the wind, sun and other environmental conditions, and helps to speed up the skin's renewal process.

Essential oils make marvellous moisturisers when blended with a suitable base oil which is appropriate to the skin type. Oils suitable as a base are:

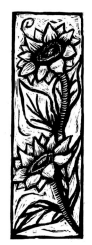

| SKIN TYPE | BASE OIL |
|---|---|
| NORMAL SKIN | *Almond, hazelnut or apricot kernel oil, with a small amount of jojoba or carrot oil.* |
| DRY SKIN | *Almond, avocado, wheat germ or olive oil, with a small amount of jojoba, carrot or evening primrose oil.* |
| OILY SKIN | *Almond, apricot kernel or grapeseed oil, with a small amount of evening primrose or carrot oil.* |
| SENSITIVE SKIN | *Apricot kernel, sunflower and safflower oil, with a small amount of jojoba oil.* |
| PROBLEM SKIN | *Soya oil, with a small amount of jojoba oil.* |
| MATURE SKIN | *Almond, hazelnut or apricot kernel oil, with a small amount of carrot and evening primrose oil.* |

The moisturiser recipe is as follows:

*30 ml (1 fl oz) of selected base oil*
*5 drops of selected additional oil (with the exception of jojoba — add 5 ml [⅛ fl oz])*
*essential oils (choose oils appropriate for your skin type from the list on page 87)*

Blend all the oils together, shaking to ensure a thorough mix, and store in an airtight, amber-coloured glass bottle. Use within two months.

Apply to facial skin after cleansing and toning, massaging gently into the skin. Leave for a few minutes, then wipe off any excess oil with a soft, clean cloth or tissue.

| SKIN TYPE | ESSENTIAL OILS |
|-----------|----------------|
| NORMAL | *20 drops rose, 5 drops lavender, 3 drops chamomile, 2 drops neroli* |
| DRY | *15 drops rose, 5 drops sandalwood, 5 drops neroli, 5 drops geranium* |
| OILY | *15 drops geranium, 10 drops lemon, 5 drops juniper* |
| SENSITIVE | *20 drops rose, 5 drops lavender, 3 drops neroli, 2 drops jasmine* |
| PROBLEM | *2 drops lavender, 1 drop lemon, 1 drop chamomile* |
| MATURE | *10 drops neroli, 5 drops rose, 5 drops frankincense, 5 drops lavender* |

## NECK MOISTURISING OIL

Each night after cleansing and toning, apply the following moisturising oil. Leave it on for two minutes, then wipe off any excess oil with a soft, clean cloth.

*35 ml (1 fl oz) jojoba oil*
*10 ml (⅓ fl oz) avocado oil*
*5 ml (⅙ fl oz) wheat germ oil*
*15 drops rose essential oil*
*10 drops carrot oil*
*5 drops neroli essential oil*

Prepare and store as for moisturiser recipe (see page 86).

# *Wrinkles*

Wrinkles are inevitable and they are something we should all accept gracefully. However, they can be prevented from occurring too soon or becoming unsightly if extra attention is given to those areas around the eyes and sides of the mouth. (See also *Eye Care*, page 90).

When applying a moisturiser, dab it gently on with your fingertips. Never drag at the delicate skin around the eyes. The same applies when removing make-up: use an oil such as almond or apricot kernel to float it off rather than rub it off.

Avoid prolonged exposure to the sun, wear a good pair of sunglasses when out-of-doors, keep your facial expression relaxed as much as possible, and make sure your diet includes sufficient protein and vitamins.

## ANTI-WRINKLE MOISTURISER
*20 ml (⅔ fl oz) almond oil*
*15 ml (½ fl oz) apricot kernel oil*
*15 ml (½ fl oz) wheat germ oil*
*10 drops geranium essential oil*
*5 drops neroli essential oil*
*2 drops chamomile essential oil*

Prepare and store as for moisturiser recipe (see page 86).

# Facial Massage Oils

The following blends are especially formulated for use at night after cleansing. Massage gently into the face as directed in *Self Facial Massage* in Chapter Four (see page 74).

Prepare the base oil as follows:

*20 ml (⅔ fl oz) almond oil*
*5 ml (⅙ fl oz) avocado oil*
*5 ml (⅙ fl oz) wheat germ oil*
*selected essential oils*

Mix all the oils together thoroughly, adding the essential oils last.

| SKIN TYPE | ESSENTIAL OILS |
|---|---|
| NORMAL SKIN | *6 drops lavender, 3 drops frankincense, 3 drops geranium, 1½ drops jasmine* |
| DRY SKIN | *4 drops rose, 4 drops sandalwood, 2 drops chamomile, 2 drops neroli* |
| OILY SKIN | *5 drops lemongrass, 4 drops lavender, 3 drops geranium* |

# Acne

Although acne is considered a teenage affliction, it can continue to be a problem beyond adolescence. It is a result of chronic inflammation of the sebaceous glands, which causes thickened sebum (oil) to mix with dead skin cells and grime, and so blocks the mouth of the pores and forms spots. Stress and anxiety can also accelerate this condition, putting into train a vicious cycle of worry which in turn only causes more spots, which only cause further worry.

The use of essential oils combined with a good diet, incorporating plenty of fresh vegetables, fruit and wholegrain foods, will get your skin off to a good start and help to maintain a clear complexion. Remember, the benefits of natural remedies and a good diet are cumulative.

Commence your skin care routine with the various preparations formulated for acne found under Cleansing (see page 78), Toning (see page 84) and Moisturising (see page 86). In addition to using the acne preparations, here are some tips for a sensible routine to help control acne:

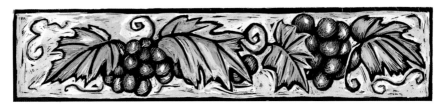

✳ *Avoid too much stress — it can aggravate acne.*

✳ *Wash skin two or three times a day with soap formulated to deal with oily skin or acne. Then cleanse with an appropriate cleanser.*

✳ *Once a week, deep-cleanse with a face mask.*

✳ *After cleansing your face, apply a tonic formulated for acne.*

✳ *Do not pick at blemishes. You will spread them and also cause scarring.*

✳ *Treat trouble spots with an acne cream, preferably one that is based on herbs rather than harsh chemicals.*

✳ *Make-up puffs, sponges or brushes that touch your face should be sterilised after use, or thrown out.*

✳ *Dirty make-up must go.*

✳ *When using make-up or creams, extract as much as you think you need and put it onto a clean saucer. Use a clean spatula for extracting creams. (At no time should you touch the contents of any tube or jar, otherwise you will contaminate it.)*

✳ *Use the saucer like an artist's palette. When you have finished, throw away any excess make-up, wipe the saucer clean, and then wash it in hot water and soap.*

✳ *Clean cottonwool is the best way to apply make-up. If you use an eye shadow brush, wash it in hot soapy water.*

✳ *Hair hanging over your face tends to aggravate acne.*

✳ *Ensure a good calcium intake. Dolomite tablets are excellent as they contain the correct balance of calcium and magnesium.*

# Eye Care

The skin under the eye is very thin and delicate, and care should be taken when removing make-up. Use a very fine oil, such as apricot kernel or almond, to remove it so that it floats off.

After cleansing, it is important to tone this tissue to ensure that the skin retains its elasticity. Gently pat elder flower water onto the skin surrounding the eye. Avoid an overgenerous application, as this will only cause stinging.

### ELDER FLOWER WATER

*1 teaspoon dried elder flowers*
*300 ml (10 fl oz) boiling water*

Place the flowers in a ceramic bowl, cover with boiling water and allow to steep until cool. Strain through muslin cloth and bottle.

This infusion will last up to 7 days if it is kept in the refrigerator, provided its container has been sterilised. Check daily to ensure that it is still usable. If it begins to smell off, do not use it. You can extend the flower water's keeping qualities by adding 3 to 4 drops simple tincture of benzoin. After toning it is important to moisturise the eye area with essential oils. They can be dabbed on gently with the fingertips around the eye area.

## Moisturising with Essential Oils

Used regularly, essential oils can help to diminish the creasing that occurs around the eyes. They will not eliminate it altogether and bring back your lost youth, but they will certainly smooth out those tiny cracks and crevices. Use only a very light and fine oil as the base, such as apricot kernel, and add the minimum amount of essential oils. Do not exceed the recommended quantities which follow.

### YOUNG SKIN

*20 ml (⅔ fl oz) apricot kernel oil*
*10 ml (⅕ fl oz) hazelnut oil*
*3 drops carrot oil*
*3 drops chamomile essential oil*

Blend all the oils together thoroughly and store in an airtight, amber-coloured glass bottle. Use within two months.

To use, gently dab a little oil around the eye area with the fingertips.

### MATURE SKIN
*20 ml (⅔ fl oz) apricot kernel oil*
*10 ml (⅓ fl oz) hazelnut oil*
*15 drops jojoba oil*
*9 drops carrot oil*
*3 drops lavender essential oil*
*3 drops neroli essential oil*

Prepare and use as for *Young Skin.*

# *Lips*

Lips can suffer from the harshness of the elements, with dry winds and sun leaving them dry, chapped and cracked. Lips look and feel their best when they are soft and smooth, and they need softening and protecting as regularly as the rest of your face does.

A medicated and moisturising lip gloss will keep your lips moist and supple, and will also soothe and repair them.

### MEDICATED LIP GLOSS
*10 g (⅓ oz) beeswax*
*5 g (⅙ oz) anhydrous lanolin*
*55 ml (2 fl oz) almond oil*
*5 ml (⅙ fl oz) jojoba oil*
*5 ml (⅙ fl oz) wheat germ oil*
*40 ml (1½ fl oz) rosewater*
*5 drops carrot oil*
*5 drops chamomile essential oil*
*5 drops rose essential oil*

Melt the beeswax and lanolin in a double saucepan (enamel or stainless steel) over a medium heat. When completely liquid, stir in prewarmed almond, jojoba and wheat germ oils and rosewater, until well blended. (To prewarm oils, add them and the rosewater to a saucepan and gently warm over a low heat.) Remove from heat, pour into a ceramic bowl, add the carrot oil and essential oils and beat until cool. Store in a sterilised glass jar. Use as required.

### C OLD S ORES

Add a drop of geranium essential oil to the tip of a cotton bud and gently dab the affected area. Repeat this procedure every day until the condition has eased. Alternatively, replace the essential oils in the *Medicated Lip Gloss* recipe (see page 91) with the following:

*4 drops geranium essential oil*
*4 drops tea tree essential oil*
*2 drops chamomile essential oil*

### S ORE AND C RACKED L IPS

Prepare the base as for *Medicated Lip Gloss* (see page 91), then add the following essential oils:

*5 drops lavender essential oil*
*5 drops neroli essential oil*

# *Body Oils*

Pampering your body with essential oils is a luxury everyone can enjoy. However, natural skin care preparations alone will not give your body that healthy glow.

Used regularly after a bath or shower, body oils will moisturise your skin, and also give it a golden sheen that will make you look and feel great.

Toning up your skin with a body oil is an excellent supplement to a healthy exercise program. A body oil based on essential oils enhances relaxation, circulation, muscle tone and a general feeling of wellbeing.

Apply the formula that suits your skin type as directed in Chapter Four, *Self Massage* (see page 74).

### N ORMAL S KIN

*20 ml (⅔ fl oz) almond oil*
*8 drops lavender essential oil*
*6 drops rose essential oil*
*4 drops neroli essential oil*
*2 drops chamomile essential oil*

Blend all the oils together thoroughly in a medicine glass or ceramic eggcup. This blend will be sufficient for one complete body application.

### DRY SKIN

*20 ml (⅔ fl oz) almond oil*
*8 drops patchouli essential oil*
*6 drops rose essential oil*
*4 drops geranium essential oil*
*2 drops carrot oil*

Prepare and use as for *Normal Skin* (see page 92).

### OILY SKIN

*20 ml (⅔ fl oz) almond oil*
*10 drops lemon essential oil*
*6 drops geranium essential oil*
*4 drops sandalwood essential oil*

Prepare and use as for *Normal Skin* (see page 92).

### SENSITIVE SKIN

*20 ml (⅔ fl oz) almond oil*
*15 drops rose essential oil*
*3 drops geranium essential oil*
*2 drops chamomile essential oil*

Prepare and use as for *Normal Skin* (see page 92).

### BLEMISHED SKIN

*20 ml (⅔ fl oz) almond oil*
*8 drops geranium essential oil*
*6 drops lavender essential oil*
*6 drops chamomile essential oil*

Prepare and use as for *Normal Skin* (see page 92).

### MATURE SKIN

*20 ml (⅔ fl oz) almond oil*
*12 drops rose essential oil*
*6 drops neroli essential oil*
*2 drops frankincense essential oil*

Prepare and use as for *Normal Skin* (see page 92).

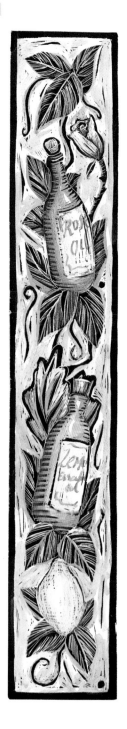

### DEODORISING BODY OIL

A certain skin type, diet, or an underlying hormonal or physiological reason, can cause a person to suffer from profuse perspiration. Usually this overactivity of the sweat glands is accompanied by an unpleasant and offensive odour. If you are prone to this condition, a deodorising body oil, applied after a bath or shower will help to keep you feeling fragrant and fresh.

Massage this oil all over the body as directed in Chapter Four, *Self Massage* (see page 74):

> *20 ml (⅔ fl oz) almond oil*
> *13 drops lavender essential oil*
> *5 drops bergamot essential oil*
> *2 drops neroli essential oil*

Prepare and use as for *Normal Skin* body oil (see page 92).

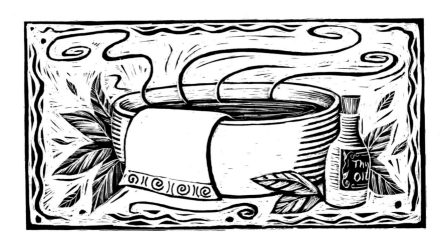

# *Body Splashes*

Body splashes are invigorating and refreshing water-based toilet waters or skin colognes. They can be liberally splashed or sprayed on, and they are ideal for use on hot summer days and nights. When you are feeling sticky and uncomfortable, their delightful tang and scent will give your spirits a lift, making you feel fresh and cool.

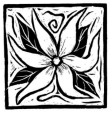

## INVIGORATING SUMMER SPLASH
*10 drops lavender essential oil*
*10 drops lime essential oil*
*5 drops grapefruit essential oil*
*5 drops lemon essential oil*
*100 ml (3½ fl oz) high proof vodka*
*500 ml (16 fl oz) distilled water*

Dissolve the essential oils in the vodka, then blend with the distilled water. Allowed to stand in an airtight glass bottle for at least 48 hours, then drip through filter paper.

## LEMON DELIGHT
*25 ml (1 fl oz) lemon essential oil*
*6 ml (⅕ fl oz) orange essential oil*
*4 ml lemongrass essential oil*
*500 ml (16 fl oz) high proof vodka*
*500 ml (16 fl oz) distilled water*

Dissolve the essential oils in the vodka, blend with the distilled water, and allow the mixture to stand for a month. Drip through filter paper and store in a tightly sealed bottle.

## CITRUS SPLASH
*1.5 ml mandarin essential oil*
*1.5 ml orange essential oil*
*10 drops lemon essential oil*
*5 drops grapefruit essential oil*
*70 ml (2½ fl oz) high proof vodka*
*430 ml (13½ fl oz) distilled water*

Prepare as for *Lemon Delight* .

# Breasts

Although the shape and size of the breasts differ from woman to woman, and are governed by many factors such as age, obesity and weight reduction, it is still important to tone and firm the pectoral muscles and to keep breast skin smooth and healthy. Essential oils are helpful here, and should be used after a bath or shower, when the skin is still warm and slightly moist. Massage with the fingers and palms, using small circular movements inwards from the outer sides of each breast, and then upwards from below each breast. Maintain strong firm strokes, pressing upwards over the nipples and up to just under the chin.

Exercising, by imitating the breast stroke movement out of water, and by pushing against the hands when they are placed at chin level with the elbows stuck out either side, is beneficial. This will strengthen the pectoral muscles and improve breast tone by keeping the fibrous tissue supple.

### BREAST MASSAGE OIL
*30 ml (1 fl oz) grapeseed oil*
*6 drops carrot oil*
*12 drops lemongrass essential oil*
*5 drops geranium essential oil*
*4 drops fennel essential oil*
*3 drops sage essential oil*

Blend all oils together thoroughly and use immediately after a bath or shower. Store any excess oil in an airtight, amber-coloured glass bottle and use within two months. This treatment should be applied every day.

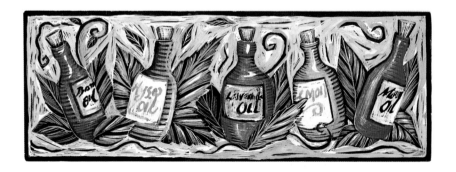

# Arms, Legs and Feet

## Arms

Regular massage and exfoliation of the arms is very important. Massaging with a lotion based on essential oils will improve the skin's elasticity, while exfoliation with a loofah mitt or friction glove will help to improve circulation and rid the skin of dead, clogging cells.

If you do not have a loofah or friction mitt handy, you can exfoliate body skin by adding 2 tablespoons of medium oatmeal and 2 tablespoons of dried chamomile flowers to a bath bag. Simply place the ingredients on a square piece of muslin, draw up the sides and tie with a piece of ribbon. Oatmeal is a well-known skin softener and, as you rub your skin, you will actually feel the impurities and rough skin float away in the bath water.

The best time to exfoliate your skin is when you are relaxing in your evening bath. Afterwards, massage the following lotion into your skin:

### ARM LOTION
*120 ml (4 fl oz) almond oil*
*20 ml (²/₅ fl oz) jojoba oil*
*80 ml (2½ fl oz) glycerine*
*20 ml (²/₅ fl oz) aloe vera juice*
*1 teaspoon lemon juice*
*6 drops chamomile essential oil*
*4 drops pumpkin oil*

Combine all ingredients in an airtight, amber-coloured glass bottle, and shake until well blended. Store in a cool place away from direct sunlight.

Use lotion generously, massaging well into the skin, and moving from the wrists upwards. Maintain firm strokes, and keep massaging until all traces of the lotion have disappeared.

## Legs

Thigh flab and cellulite are both terms used to describe the ugly rippled bulges which can appear on the insides and backs of thighs. Swimming, cycling and yoga exercises are all ideal for keeping the leg muscles trim.

Friction massage with a loofah or friction mitt during a warm bath is good for accelerating cell metabolism and improving the circulation.

Coarse sea salt on the loofah helps to improve skin colour, and is excellent for clearing flaky skin and spots. Always massage upwards, in the direction of the heart.

The lower legs can also suffer from the same problems. As with the thighs, exfoliating the skin with a loofah should be done several times a week at bathtime. For more stubborn areas, massage with coarse sea salt or an oatmeal bath bag, rinse off thoroughly, and pat dry with a towel. Then massage the legs with the following oil, making rotating movements on the cellulite areas:

## LEG MASSAGE OIL

*15 ml (½ fl oz) almond oil*
*2 drops jojoba oil*
*2 drops carrot oil*
*7 drops cypress essential oil*
*3 drops juniper essential oil*
*2 drops lavender essential oil*

Combine all the oils in a medicine glass or ceramic eggcup, mixing until thoroughly blended.

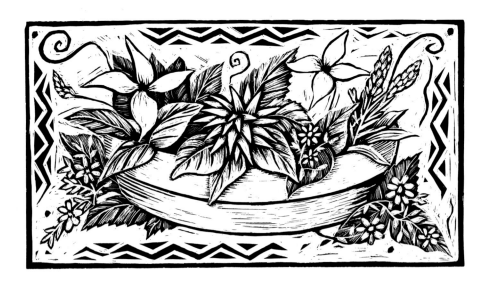

# *Feet*

Feet are often the most neglected part of the body, yet within the average lifetime they will walk the equivalent of four times around the world. Tired feet make a tired-looking face, so take time out to give yours the attention they deserve and treat them with care.

At the end of a busy day, the therapeutic footbath in Chapter One (see page 12) and the *Quick Foot Massage* in Chapter Four (see page 65) will work wonders for tired and aching feet. If you have not got the time for a separate footbath, rub rosemary essential oil or diluted apple cider vinegar into your feet, massaging for about 5 minutes, before you take a bath.

For those in a particular hurry, a quick soak in a basin of water to which has been added a few drops of peppermint essential oil will soon perk you up. It is extremely refreshing, and marvellous after a long day of shopping. For those of you who enjoy a lot of walking, give your feet a quick soak in a footbath using geranium oil before you set out. It strengthens the skin and improves elasticity and circulation, and helps to prevent the occurrence of blisters.

## SOOTHING FOOTBATH

To a basin of warm water, add the following:

*1 tablespoon sea salt*
*2 drops hyssop essential oil*
*1 drop rosemary essential oil*
*1 drop bay leaf essential oil*
*1 drop rose essential oil*

Stir in the sea salt until it dissolves, add the essential oils, mixing them in well with your hand, and then soak your feet. After 10 minutes, revive your feet with a quick dip in a basin of cold water, and then return them to the footbath. Continue doing this as long as the water is warm, finishing with a cold dip. After your footbath, massage the following lotion into your feet, taking time to massage the toes well:

*15 ml (½ fl oz) almond oil*
*5 ml (⅙ fl oz) avocado oil*
*6 drops rosemary essential oil*

Blend the oils in a small, airtight, amber-coloured glass bottle. Store in a cool place.

Follow these simple guidelines to keep your feet in tiptop condition:

❊ *Let your feet breathe. Walk barefoot as often as possible to let your feet recover from the confinement of shoes.*

❊ *When out-of-doors, and during leisure time, wear sensible footwear: flat-heeled, comfortable, open leather shoes or sandals.*

❊ *Refrain from wearing nylon stockings unless it is absolutely essential.*

❊ *Treat your feet with care and exercise them daily. A simple and quick foot exercise: to help firm muscles and recover from the confinement of shoes, gently stretch the arch and curl toes underneath. Hold this position and count to 10. Do this 3 times with each foot whenever you are sitting down.*

❊ *Shop for shoes in the afternoon, for your feet will swell during the day.*

❊ *Make sure your shoes are at least 2.5 cm (¾ in) longer than your toes. Choose shoes with heels less than 5 cm (2 in) high.*

❊ *Avoid wearing the same pair of shoes every day.*

❊ *Do not buy plastic shoes. Instead, choose leather or fabric which will allow feet to breathe.*

❊ *Avoid wearing tight boots for long periods, as they tend to restrict circulation.*

❊ *Give your feet a regular pedicure, and always cut the toenails straight across.*

❊ *For dry skin on your feet, wash with a mixture of 1 tablespoon of bran and 3 tablespoons of strong chamomile infusion (about 3 level teaspoons of chamomile to 300 ml [10 fl oz] of boiling water). Rinse, wipe dry, and then moisturise with the foot lotion on page 99.*

❊ *Soften very hard skin on the soles of the feet or the backs of the heels by massaging with equal quantities of olive oil and cider vinegar. Smooth daily with a natural pumice stone.*

❊ *Prevent foot odour and excessive perspiration by ensuring that you have sufficient silica in your diet. Include barley, kelp, garlic, onions, parsley, lettuce and celery.*

❊ *Wear socks made from natural fibres because they breathe, whereas synthetics will encourage perspiration.*

# CHAPTER SIX

# Essential Hair Care

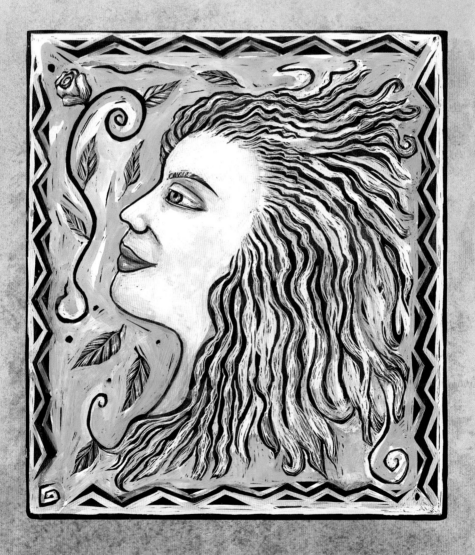

The condition of your hair is a fairly good indication of your general state of health. An unruly tangle of limp, lifeless hair affects both your looks and the way you feel. Shiny, bouncy hair is an enviable asset that everyone notices.

If you feel even slightly out-of-sorts it is surprising how quickly your hair will lose its sheen and body. Maintaining a balanced diet is essential for healthy, beautiful hair, as hair needs vitamin B complex, vitamin A, calcium, silica, iron, zinc, protein and unsaturated oils or fatty acids.

Although diet is the foundation of healthy hair, the regular use of essential oils will also help to give it a natural beauty. Essential oils will not affect the natural colour of your hair. In combination with certain herbs, these oils will nourish and moisturise both your hair and scalp.

To maintain the healthy lustre and body that is so important to your hair, try the gentle cleansing action of a natural aroma-shampoo and conditioner. There is nothing more refreshing than to wash your hair with a home-made shampoo from nature, and these products will also keep your hair shiny, healthy and manageable.

However, unlike their commercial counterparts, shampoos made in the kitchen contain no synthetics, detergents or chemicals, in particular phosphates. They will not lather up like the store-bought varieties, but they will leave your hair squeaky-clean and in excellent condition. For newcomers to natural shampoos, it will actually feel as though you are oiling your hair when you begin to wash it. However, just keep massaging the shampoo into the scalp and hair, then rinse. You will immediately notice the difference: fresh, clean hair.

## Nourishing and Moisturising

Your scalp can dry out just like your facial skin, leaving you with flaky skin and dandruff. This condition can be remedied with the regular use of a mildly antiseptic pre-wash conditioner that will stimulate, purify, nourish and moisturise your scalp.

### PRE-WASH CONDITIONER
This blend has a base of almond oil, which is similar to your own scalp oil and acts as an excellent emollient, protecting your skin by replacing natural surface oils and preventing roughness and chapping.

*80 ml (2½ fl oz) almond oil*
*10 ml (⅓ fl oz) avocado oil*
*10 ml (⅓ fl oz) wheat germ oil*
*4 drops rosemary essential oil*
*1 drop peppermint essential oil*

Thoroughly blend all the oils and store in an airtight, amber-coloured glass bottle away from heat. Use within four months.

Massage this conditioner into your scalp whenever it needs extra conditioning and dry flaky skin is evident.

### HAIR THAT TANGLES

For dry hair that tangles when wet, pre-condition with a few drops of a half-and-half mixture of rosemary and lavender essential oils. Massage well into the scalp about half an hour before shampooing.

# Types of Hair

## Normal Hair

This is neither dry nor greasy, and it is always shiny and easy to manage. However, normal hair can still turn dry or greasy if dandruff develops.

Essential oils suitable for a base shampoo for normal hair are lavender, rosemary, lemon and geranium.

## Oily Hair

Oily hair is often the result of overactive sebaceous glands, and it usually looks unwashed and lanky. However, continual washing actually exacerbates the problem, especially if harsh detergent-based shampoos are used. Shampooing less often, and with a natural shampoo, will help to add life to greasy hair.

Essential oils to include in a shampoo for oily hair are rosemary, lemon, lavender, basil, thyme and yarrow.

## Fair Hair

Oils to use are chamomile, lavender, lemon and rosemary.

## Dark Hair

Oils to use are rosemary, sage, lemon, lavender and carrot.

## Fragile Hair

This condition is usually the result of over-abuse of the hair, including too many perms, the use of heated rollers and hair dryers, teasing, colours and gels. To correct the problem, hair has to be treated gently to encourage new and stronger growth.

Essential oils that can be used in a shampoo for fragile hair are carrot, chamomile, lavender, calendula, thyme and sandalwood.

## Dandruff

Food allergies and sugary diets can often promote dandruff. Watch your diet and try to see if there is any correlation between what you have eaten in the last 48 hours and how bad your scalp is.

Effective essential oils to include in an anti-dandruff shampoo base are rosemary, nutmeg, lemon, thyme, basil, peppermint, lavender and sage.

# Shampoos

Since there is so much variation in hair type, colour and texture, it is important to use the correct shampoo for your individual needs. Choose from any of the oils singly or in combination, specified for your particular hair type (under *Types of Hair*, see page 103) and add them to the base shampoo recipe.

### AROMA-SHAMPOO BASE

This is an excellent shampoo that will cleanse, moisturise and nourish the hair and scalp.

*30 ml (1 fl oz) almond oil*
*30 ml (1 fl oz) castor oil*
*180 ml (6 fl oz) herbal infusion (see instructions which follow)*
*6 drops essential oil(s) of choice*

Combine all the ingredients in a suitable bottle, shake well, and store for future use. Shake vigorously before using. Massage shampoo into scalp and hair for 1 to 2 minutes, then rinse thoroughly.

### HERBAL INFUSION

Prepare the infusion by adding 2 teaspoons of dried herbs (chosen from the list on page 105) to a ceramic bowl and cover with 300 ml

(10 fl oz) of boiling water. Steep until cold, strain through muslin cloth, and add required amount to base recipe.

For a stronger infusion steep for 12 hours before straining.

## *Shampoo Herbs*

Choose from the following herbs, according to your hair type. Prepare as previously directed for the *Herbal Infusion* above.

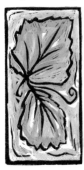

FAIR HAIR • *Chamomile — has a lightening effect and is healing to scalp irritations.*

DARK HAIR • *Rosemary or sage.*

DANDRUFF • *Nettle, parsley, peppermint, rosemary and thyme. A combination of thyme, rosemary and peppermint will control dandruff and act as a scalp and hair tonic.*

OILY HAIR • *Sage, yarrow, rosemary and lime (linden) flowers.*

HEALING • *Chamomile, parsley, rosemary and peppermint.*

### AFTER-SHAMPOO RINSE

An after-shampoo rinse gives added health and shine to your hair, removes any remaining shampoo residue, and helps to balance the scalp's pH level. Choose from the shampoo herbs appropriate to your needs. Prepare as previously directed for the *Herbal Infusion* above.

After washing your hair, rinse thoroughly with clean water and then pour over the herbal rinse. Repeat this procedure several times, each time massaging the rinse well into your hair and scalp with the tips of the fingers. On the final rinse, continue to massage the scalp for about 2 minutes.

## *Conditioners*

Continual shampooing can strip the natural oils from your scalp and hair. Your scalp becomes dry and flaky and your hair will begin to look dull and lifeless. Essential oils can help to remedy these problems. Here are some tips:

※ *After shampooing, take 1 or 2 drops of either rosemary or lavender essential oil, or a combination of both, and rub between the palms of the hands, then lightly apply over your wet hair.*

※ *A few drops of rosemary oil rubbed into the scalp after washing stimulates the circulation of the blood and makes an excellent skin conditioner.*

✳ *For brittle hair, prepare a blend made up of two-thirds rosemary essential oil and one-third olive oil. Rub between the palms of the hand and apply to wet hair.*

Alternatively, pre-condition with olive oil or castor oil. Rub a small quantity into your scalp and hair and then wrap your head in a warm wet towel for 30 minutes, putting a shower cap over the towel to keep the warmth in. Shampoo, and then give hair a final rinse with water containing vinegar or lemon juice.

## MONTHLY PROTEIN CONDITIONER

This quick and easy-to-make protein conditioner can be applied to the hair once a month. It will keep hair shiny and healthy, giving it life and bounce that everyone notices.

*20 ml (⅔ fl oz) almond oil*
*20 ml (⅔ fl oz) wheat germ oil*
*2 drops rosemary essential oil*
*1 drop lavender essential oil*
*20 ml (⅔ fl oz) glycerine*
*10 ml (⅓ fl oz) cider vinegar*
*1 egg*

Blend all the oils with glycerine, add the vinegar and then beat thoroughly with the egg. After shampooing, massage conditioner thoroughly into the hair, cover with a shower cap and leave for 30 minutes. Shampoo out, rinse with clean water and then apply a herbal after-shampoo rinse (see page 105).

# Dandruff

After washing your hair, rinse clean with the following after-shampoo rinse, massaging it well into the scalp and hair.

## ANTI-DANDRUFF RINSE

*2 teaspoons dried rosemary*
*2 teaspoons dried thyme*
*1 teaspoon dried peppermint*
*1 tablespoon dried chamomile for fair hair or dried sage for dark hair*
*2 tablespoons lemon juice*
*4 drops rosemary essential oil*

Place the selected herbs in a ceramic bowl, pour in boiling water, cover and steep overnight. Strain through muslin cloth, and then add the lemon juice and rosemary oil. Store in an airtight bottle in the refrigerator until needed. Shake well before use.

After washing your hair, rinse it thoroughly with clean water and then pour over the herbal rinse. Repeat several times.

## ANTI-DANDRUFF CONDITIONING OIL

Use this treatment weekly. To apply, wet hair thoroughly and massage *Conditioning Oil* well into the scalp and hair with fingertips for about 2 minutes. Rinse clean.

*1 teaspoon dried rosemary*
*300 ml (10 fl oz) boiling water*
*30 ml (1 fl oz) almond oil*
*30 ml (1 fl oz) castor oil*
*10 drops rosemary essential oil*
*10 drops chamomile essential oil*

Put dried rosemary in a ceramic bowl, add boiling water, cover and steep for 12 hours. Strain and blend 180 ml (6 fl oz) of this infusion with the oils. Store in an old shampoo bottle. Any excess infusion can be added to your bath or drunk as a herbal tea, and stored in the refrigerator for up to 7 days.

## VINEGAR RINSE

This is an overnight treatment that dandruff will respond to very well.

*5 drops rosemary essential oil*
*4 drops thyme essential oil*
*1 drop peppermint essential oil*
*20 ml (⅔ fl oz) apple cider vinegar*
*30 ml (1 fl oz) distilled water*

Dissolve the essential oils in the cider vinegar and then blend thoroughly with the distilled water. Store in an airtight glass bottle.

Use this lotion each night until the condition clears. Massage a teaspoonful well into the scalp, but not your hair, with the fingertips for about 2 to 3 minutes.

# CHAPTER SEVEN

# Just for Women

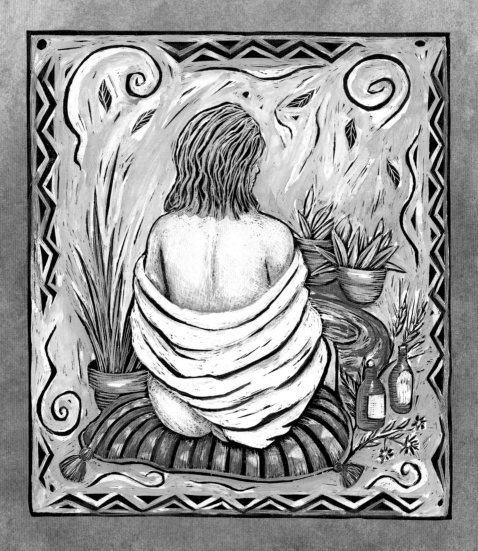

# *Menstrual Problems*

No two women are alike in the way their monthly period affects them. For many, it is accompanied by unpleasant side effects, such as uterine cramp, muscular and abdominal pains, water retention, sore breasts, headaches, fatigue, irritability and depression. Some women suffer from profuse menstruation, while others have a scanty menstrual flow. If your general state of health is good there is usually no need to concern yourself about a scanty period. However, it is advisable to include the following in your diet: fresh grated beetroot, barley, green beans, strawberries, lettuce, brown rice and soya beans. Dietary modification will also assist women who are prone to heavy periods, and the following should be included: carrots, lentils, parsley and ginger.

Certain essential oils are also useful in easing the various problems and helping to alleviate discomfort. However, with conditions such as continuous water retention, pain and irritability, and other long term symptoms, medical attention is required.

Essential oils are delightful to use in any body preparation and, quite apart from their therapeutic qualities, their pleasing fragrance will leave you feeling special.

When using essential oils to help relieve menstrual problems, use them in moderation and only as a support. They can be applied as a body rub or added to your bath. Do not attempt to use them internally.

Oils to use singly or in combination are: rose, oregano, marjoram, melissa, geranium, nutmeg, bergamot, clary sage, rosemary, cypress, chamomile and myrrh. For a body rub, add 30 drops of essential oil to 30 ml (1 fl oz) of almond oil and store in an airtight, amber-coloured glass bottle. Add a teaspoon of this mixture to a warm bath, or add 8 to 10 drops of neat essential oil to your bath each day during the period.

To apply the body rub, adopt the self-massage techniques described in Chapter Four, page 74. Concentrate only on the abdomen, hips and lower back, extending down between the buttocks but keeping well clear of the anus.

The following blends are general formulas and may not suit every individual. You can mix and blend any of the suggested oils (or use them singly) in the same ratio, until you find a formula unique to your individual needs.

## A BDOMINAL  P AIN  AND  C RAMPS

*30 ml (1 fl oz) almond oil*
*12 drops chamomile essential oil*
*9 drops cypress essential oil*
*9 drops clary sage essential oil*

For cramping of the female organs, relief can be obtained by rubbing an oregano oil blend into the lower parts of the body. In addition, linseed tea, taken as needed, can help to give relief from the pain. To make the tea, add 2 tablespoons of linseeds to 750 ml (24 fl oz) of boiling water, add a pinch of cinnamon, the juice of half a lemon and a teaspoon of brown sugar. Simmer over a gentle heat for about 20 minutes, and strain before use.

## S EVERE  M ENSTRUAL  P AIN

For severe menstrual pain, take 15 drops of 'spirit of balm' in a glass of water every half hour.

Spirit of balm is made from the tangy lemon-scented leaves of *Melissa officinalis* (lemon balm). It grows quickly from seed, is self-seeding, and will grow almost anywhere. You can make your own spirit of balm blend as follows:

*1 cup (155 g/5 oz) fresh lemon balm leaves, tightly packed*
*750 ml (24 fl oz) high proof vodka*
*750 ml (24 fl oz) distilled water*

Put all the ingredients in a glass jar, seal with an airtight lid and leave in a warm place for several days. Strain mixture, drip through filter paper and store in an airtight glass bottle. Use as directed above.

## P RE - MENSTRUAL  T ENSION

Use selected essential oils in a body rub and/or add to your bath. Those oils which are particularly useful are rose, bergamot, geranium, clary sage, cypress, nutmeg and chamomile.

A suggested blend could be:

*30 ml (1 fl oz) almond oil*
*12 drops rose essential oil*
*9 drops chamomile essential oil*
*9 drops bergamot essential oil*

# Pregnancy

For many women, pregnancy causes changes and upheavals in the body that result in considerable discomfort and stress. Minor problems such as backache, swollen legs, reversal of skin condition (oily to dry or vice versa), lack of skin tone, morning sickness and insomnia can be aided by the use of essential oils, moderate exercise and dietary modification.

Cleanse and moisturise the skin as directed in Chapter Five (see page 78), and include plenty of fresh fruit and vegetables (in particular broad beans, climbing and dwarf beans, and peas), wholemeal cereal products, poultry and fish in the diet. Avoid red meat as much as possible, or completely abstain from it. Exercise daily by walking and/or swimming until it no longer feels comfortable. Only undertake an exercise program after consultation with your medical practitioner.

## Backache and Swollen Legs

My wife still maintains there was no joy at all while she was carrying, and some of the lesser joys of pregnancy are the inevitable backache, swollen legs and tiredness that overtake your whole body.

The uplifting qualities of essential oils will help to ease the aches and lethargy, soothe the spirits and put the world back in perspective. Add them to a warm bath, or include in a soothing and relaxing body rub.

For a relaxing and uplifting bath which is especially beneficial for swollen legs, add 1 drop each of chamomile and lavender essential oils to the bath water once the taps are turned off and the water temperature begins to drop. Or, ask your partner to gently massage your back with the following blend each evening before retiring:

*40 ml (1½ fl oz) almond oil*
*5 ml (⅙ fl oz) avocado oil*
*5 ml (⅙ fl oz) wheat germ oil*
*8 drops geranium essential oil*
*8 drops lavender essential oil*
*4 drops chamomile essential oil*

Thoroughly blend all oils together and store in an airtight, amber-coloured glass bottle. Shake well before use.

## Morning Sickness

When carrying our first child, my wife was plagued at first with morning sickness. To overcome the problem and calm her stomach, a drop of spearmint essential oil was placed on her pillow each evening. On the floor beside the bed, I placed a bowl of boiling water to which I added 6 drops of the same essential oil.

As she slept, she inhaled the calming fragrance of the spearmint oil, reducing the possibility of nausea and morning sickness.

This same procedure was adopted with our second child right from the beginning of the pregnancy, and it was successful in preventing any symptoms of morning sickness and nausea.

## Insomnia

To relieve insomnia, try putting a drop of basil, chamomile, clary sage or lavender essential oil onto your pillow at night.

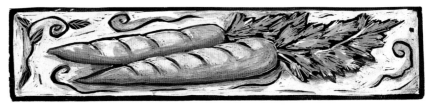

## Stretch Marks

A concern all pregnant women share is the legacy of stretch marks. To help prevent this problem it is important to maintain the tone and elasticity of the skin by regularly massaging those areas where stretch marks are likely to occur, such as the lower and upper abdomen, thighs and buttocks.

Massage any problem areas with the following oil blend, or use the formula in Chapter Four, page 61.

*40 ml (1½ fl oz) almond oil*
*5 ml (⅙ fl oz) avocado oil*
*5 ml (⅙ fl oz) wheat germ oil*
*5 drops carrot oil*
*8 drops tangerine essential oil*
*7 drops mandarin essential oil*

Thoroughly blend all oils together and store in an airtight, amber-coloured glass bottle. Shake well before use.

# Breast Care

Few women are satisfied with the shape and size of their breasts, and look for ways to change them so that they conform with the demands of current trends. While no cream can enlarge the breasts, or turn them into something they are not, it is important to look after them.

The shape and size of a woman's breasts are largely determined by inherited genes and hormone levels, and other governing factors, such as obesity. Breast shape and size are also related to the condition of the pectoral muscles which support them. Massage, and the use of essential oils, will strengthen these muscles and help to maintain muscle tone. For tips on regular care of the breasts, including massage techniques and exercise, refer to the instructions in Chapter Five, page 96.

# Cracked Nipples

This problem is more common than most people realise, and is even more likely to occur after childbirth. Apart from being extremely painful, there is also the possibility of an infection with this condition. It is therefore important to take proper care of the nipples and to prevent this condition from occurring.

Apply the *Cracked Nipple Moisturising Oil* below after a bath or shower, massaging over the whole nipple and areola area. Start with the nipples, gently massaging each one by rolling it between a well-oiled thumb and forefinger for about 2 minutes. Then continue to gently massage the areola with well-oiled fingertips, using small circular movements. The breasts can then be massaged as directed in Chapter Five (see page 96).

### CRACKED NIPPLE MOISTURISING OIL

*25 ml (1 fl oz) almond oil*
*20 ml (⅔ fl oz) apricot kernel oil*
*5 ml (⅙ fl oz) wheat germ oil*
*10 drops calendula essential oil*
*8 drops rose essential oil*
*7 drops chamomile essential oil*

Thoroughly blend all the oils together and store in an airtight, amber-coloured glass bottle.

# *Varicose Veins*

Varicose veins require professional treatment. However, in the early stages, gentle fingertip massage in the direction of the heart and compresses may be of assistance. When massaging the affected area of the legs, gentleness cannot be overemphasised: undue pressure from normal massage techniques can quite easily damage the fragile capillary walls.

Walking is also important to prevent further congestion of the veins and to keep the blood circulating. Putting your feet up for an hour each evening after a footbath is also beneficial, as is a good diet and ensuring regular bowel movements.

## FINGERTIP MASSAGE OIL
*27 ml (1 fl oz) hazelnut oil*
*5 ml wheat germ oil*
*20 drops geranium essential oil*
*10 drops cypress essential oil*

Thoroughly blend all oils together and store in an airtight, amber-coloured glass bottle. Use within 2 months.

## COMPRESS
*4 drops geranium essential oil*
*2 drops cypress essential oil*
*500 ml (16 fl oz) water*

Put the essential oils in a basin of hot water, sufficient to cover a compress. Soak the compress for 2 minutes, then squeeze it out until it stops dripping. Apply to the affected area and cover with plastic and a prewarmed towel. Leave on for at least 2 hours.

## FOOTBATH
In two basins which are large enough to hold your feet when they are stretched out, pour sufficient hot water in one and cold water in the other to reach your ankles. Add 3 to 4 drops of geranium essential oil to the hot water and 3 to 4 drops of lavender essential oil to the cold water.

Before soaking your feet give each one a preliminary massage. Do this while sitting comfortably; place one foot over your knee and press, rub and pull each toe, then knead the sole with your knuckles. Next place the fingers of both hands on the sole, and the thumbs, pointing toward the toes, on the top of the foot, and stroke down from the ankles to the toes. Now put your feet in the hot water and soak them for 5 minutes. Then soak them in the cold water for five minutes. Continue doing this as long as the hot water stays hot, then finish with a cold dip.

Remove one foot at a time, drying them and then rubbing with the following massage oil:

*27 ml (1 fl oz) hazelnut oil*
*3 ml wheat germ oil*
*12 drops geranium essential oil*
*9 drops marigold essential oil*
*9 drops cypress essential oil*

Prepare as for the *Fingertip Massage Oil* (see page 114).

# *Menopause*

Many women regard the approach of menopause with fear and see it as the beginning of a decline in the quality of their life. There is Hormone Replacement Therapy (HRT), which has received a lot of publicity of late, and is touted as being able to solve all the problems associated with this change of life. From my own observations, none of the experts can yet agree as to what physiological problems, if any, may result.

HRT is a matter of individual choice. However, good nutrition, including plenty of raw fruit and vegetables in the diet, a sufficient vitamin intake, the use of cold-pressed cooking oils and a supplement of evening primrose oil will all be beneficial. Exclude stimulants from your diet, especially tea, coffee and alcohol, and drink non-addictive herbal teas instead.

Including ginseng in your diet will provide a natural source of oestrogen. Check with your health practitioner first, since ginseng is a natural steroid. Headaches, migraine, dizziness and nausea can be treated by taking 1 small glass of fresh cucumber juice daily.

Cypress, geranium and sage essential oils included in your bath or in a daily massage oil will help with circulatory problems, such as hot flushes, day and night sweats and water retention. Blend in a 9:16:5 ratio with 30 ml (1 fl oz) of almond oil, and store in an airtight, amber-coloured glass bottle.

When massaging, always massage in the direction of the heart: for instance, from the feet to the thighs, and from the hands to the shoulders. If the whole body is affected, ask someone to massage both the front and back of your torso, and use no more than a teaspoon of oil. This should be done daily in conjunction with a warm, relaxing bath, which should be taken prior to your massage. Add 10 drops of the same oil blend to hot bath water once it has settled.

# Cellulite

Cellulite is the skin condition where fatty deposits, excess fluids and toxins become trapped under the skin, especially around the thigh area in women. It leaves hard pads of fat which look a little like the pitted marks of an orange skin.

Chapter Five deals with the exfoliation of the skin and the use of a massage oil formulated for cellulite. Although massage is one of the greatest weapons in fighting this condition, correct diet and exercise are also important. Avoid processed foods containing colourings, flavourings and preservatives. Eliminate alcohol, or at least reduce any regular consumption to a minimum, and cut down on fat, salt, seasonings and spices. If possible, wean yourself completely off all seasonings and enjoy the natural taste of food. Your diet should include lean meat, eggs, natural yoghurt, wheat germ, honey, skimmed milk, and plenty of raw fruit and vegetables, especially grapefruit, pineapple, grapes, asparagus, radishes and onions. Drink at least 8 glasses of water every day.

Exercise, especially the quality of the exercise you select, will also help combat cellulite by improving circulation and muscle tone. Avoid exercise programs which put strain on the leg muscles or jar the hips and thighs, such as running, jogging, squash, tennis or strenuous aerobic workouts. Stick to fairly brisk walking, cycling, swimming and yoga instead.

Bath water additives will also help, and can be used in conjunction with the exfoliating instructions on page 97. Blend together geranium, lemongrass and cypress oils in a 12:16:12 ratio with 40 ml (1½ fl oz) of almond oil. Store in an airtight, amber-coloured glass bottle and use within two months. Add 1 teaspoon of oil to a hot bath once the water has settled. Towel dry and then apply the massage oil as directed.

# CHAPTER EIGHT

# Creating an Aromatic Environment

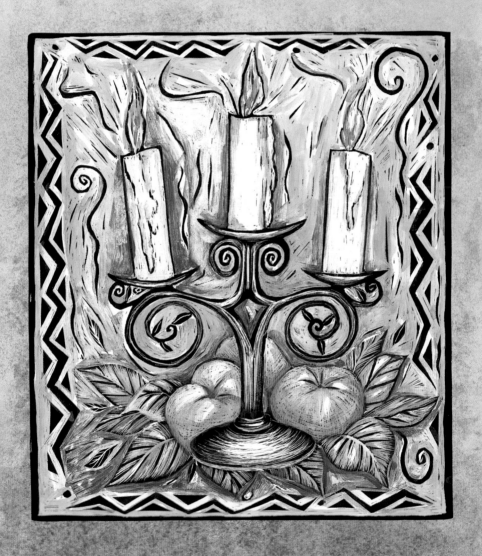

# Air Fresheners

The refreshing and aromatic properties of essential oils can be used in many different ways to keep your home fragrant and fresh. Not only will they remove stale and unwanted odours, but they will also provide protection against airborne viruses and bacteria through their antifungal and antibacterial properties.

An air freshener spray is one of the simplest ways in which you can use essential oils to perfume your home. Try just one aromatic oil or a blend of many oils that will release an immediate burst of fragrance to tease the senses, and then leave a lingering, elusive scent to keep rooms smelling fresh.

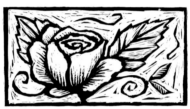

## JUDITH'S BREATH OF FRESH AIR

This is one of my wife's favourite blends.

*25 drops lavender essential oil*
*15 drops lemon essential oil*
*10 drops geranium essential oil*
*5 drops ylang-ylang essential oil*
*10 ml (⅓ fl oz) methylated spirits*
*500 ml (16 fl oz) distilled water*

Dissolve the essential oils in the methylated spirits and then blend with the distilled water. Store in a pump-spray bottle and use on a fine mist setting.

# Burning Essential Oils

Burning essential oils will kill airborne bacteria and fungi. Although any oil will impart its special fragrance, some can also be used for specific purposes. Try lavender, thyme, eucalyptus or pine for their fresh fragrance, or lavender or peppermint in a sick room as protection against bacteria.

You can burn oils singly or as a blend to create that special atmosphere. Here are some of the ways in which you can do this:

✳ *Add a few drops of essential oil to a shallow dish of warm water set on a sunny windowsill or radiator. As it evaporates, its aroma will fill the room.*

✳ *One or two drops of oil on a warm light bulb will quickly fill the room with fragrance. Place a few drops of one oil or a blend of oils in a light bulb ring, turn on the light and a gentle fragrance will waft around your home. Light bulb rings can be used on both ceiling lights and lamps and are available from most gift shops.*

✳ *For a sweet-smelling bathroom, dab a few drops of your favourite aromatic oil onto the spout of the hot tap and turn it on for a few moments to release the fragrance. The delightful aroma will fill the room for some time.*

✳ *A ceramic simmering pot, available from gift shops and some supermarkets, is an ideal way of burning particular essential oil blends. A simmering pot is a small ceramic vessel with a candle inside and a saucer for containing the fragrant mixture sitting on top. Add about 10 drops of essential oil to one cup of boiling water, preheat the saucer by burning the candle, and then three-quarters fill it with the fragrant water, topping up when required. The following blend can be used:*

### Sweet Ambrosial Blend
*3 drops bergamot essential oil*
*2 drops nutmeg essential oil*
*1 drop lavender essential oil*
*250 ml (8 fl oz) boiling water*

## Incense

For hundreds of years herbs, spices and oils have been blended and used as incense to cover up and eliminate offensive odours in the home, or burnt in religious ceremonies. Burning scents like frankincense and myrrh dates back to the time of the ancient Egyptians, and the practice still has a place in our homes today: not to mask the fetid odours of yesteryear, but to perfume the air with an enjoyable sweetness.

The following blend is delightful to use, but with a little imagination and experimentation I am sure that you will develop your own fragrances that are just as enjoyable to the senses.

## SWEET LAVENDER INCENSE

*1 tablespoon very fine sawdust*
*1 teaspoon each of dried lavender, dried rose petals and dried cloves*
*(Reduce to a powder with a pestle and mortar, and then rub through a fine wire sieve.)*
*1 teaspoon orrisroot powder*
*1 tablespoon distilled water*
*1 teaspoon gum arabic*
*3 drops lavender essential oil*
*3 drops rose essential oil*
*3 drops clove essential oil*

Thoroughly mix the sawdust with herbs, cloves and orrisroot powder, then add 1 tablespoon of water in which the gum arabic has been dissolved. Add the essential oils, blending well to ensure a thorough mix. When all the ingredients are mixed together, shape into cones and allow to dry.

Place cones on small metal dishes, or other suitable objects, and then light — the incense will smoulder, filling the room with fragrance.

For more exotic fragrances, or an aroma that is a little mysterious, experiment with your own blends by mixing different herbs, spices and oils.

# Fragrant Candles

Burning fragrant candles adds a lovely touch of warmth to a home and, unlike those scented by chemicals, naturally scented candles are very subtle and not overpowering.

Beeswax makes the best candles, but can be expensive unless you can purchase it direct from a beekeeper. Regardless, any additional expense is worth the end result.

For moulds you can use empty drink cans, milk cartons, toilet roll cylinders, yoghurt containers, and so on. Wicks can be purchased from hobby suppliers or craft shops, or you can use No. 4 knitting cotton.

Melt the wax in a double saucepan over a medium heat so that it does not burn. When it is completely liquid, add 5 ml (⅙ fl oz) of essential oil for every 500 ml (16 fl oz) of liquid wax. If you feel the scent is not strong enough, you can melt the wax again and add more essential oil.

Attach one end of the wick to a piece of plasticine, position in the centre of the bottom of the mould, and secure the other end to a pencil laid across the top. Pour in the liquid wax and allow to harden for at least 3 to 4 hours before using. Trim the wick to 1 cm (¼ in), remove the candle from the mould and discard the plasticine.

When using toilet roll cylinders as moulds, tape a circular cardboard disc to the bottom.

Make your candles to suit particular moods: stimulating, relaxing or romantic. Essential oils to choose from are:

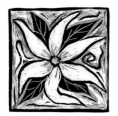

| STIMULATING | RELAXING | ROMANTIC |
|---|---|---|
| *Grapefruit* | *Geranium* | *Patchouli* |
| *Coriander* | *Sandalwood* | *Ylang-ylang* |
| *Melissa* | *Rose* | *Rose* |
| *Mandarin* | *Frankincense* | *Jasmine* |

Of course, you are not limited by these suggested oils. One of my personal favourites is the fragrance of lavender, or use a special blend of a number of different oils. Two other favourites are sandalwood and patchouli in a 4:2 ratio, or equal amounts of honeysuckle and violet essential oils. Experimenting is half the fun.

## *Perfumed Pillows and Bed Linen*

There is nothing new about perfumed bed linen. In the Middle Ages the laundresses would drape the household sheets over lavender bushes to dry and to impart their fresh, clean scent. Today we can use the magic of essential oils to perfume our sheets and make them a fragrant delight to slide between.

Add 5 drops of your chosen essential oil to the softener compartment of your washing machine. If your machine is not quite so modern, simply put a few drops of essential oil on a face washer and throw that in with the rest of your wash, or put it in the clothes drier if you use one.

A drop of essential oil on a pillowcase will tantalise the senses for a romantic interlude, or exert a soporific effect and lull you off to sleep.

Choose any of the following essential oils for a fresh, floral or romantic fragrance (see page 122).

| FRESH | FLORAL | ROMANTIC |
|-------|--------|----------|
| *Lavender* | *Geranium* | *Ylang-ylang* |
| *Bergamot* | *Neroli* | *Rose* |
| *Lemon* | *Honeysuckle* | *Jasmine* |
| *Rosemary* | *Violet* | *Musk* |

You can also use essential oils when ironing pillowcases and bed linen. Dissolve 3 to 4 ml of your chosen oil or blend of oils in 10 ml (⅓ fl oz) of methylated spirits and blend this with 500 ml (16 fl oz) of distilled water. Store in a pump-spray bottle and spray on linen, using a fine mist setting, as you iron.

For bed linen that is to be stored away, add a couple of drops of essential oil to a number of different cottonwool balls and put them in between the layers of the sheets.

# *Edible Essential Oils*

Theoretically, all essential oils are edible in minute quantities — 1 to 3 drops. However, it is not wise to start consuming different oils just because they may taste or smell good.

The most commonly used oils, especially in chocolates where a strong flavour is required, are aniseed, basil, bergamot orange (be sure that it is the edible variety), cinnamon, ginger, lemon, lime, orange, peppermint, rosemary, spearmint and nutmeg.

There are many home chocolate-making kits available, so why not give your family and friends a different taste treat? And, for those who like to partake of unusual alcoholic beverages, a drop of nutmeg oil in a Brandy Alexander is — well, only one word can describe it — yum! Different oils work best with different drinks, especially liqueurs and coffee, and are really a matter of individual taste. Have fun deciding what you like best!

A drop of peppermint essential oil added to a glass of warm water in which a little honey has been dissolved counters indigestion and nausea. It acts extremely quickly. This also works well to counteract nausea during pregnancy.

# Glossary

AMOISE • *Essential oil from the herb mugwort.*

ANHYDROUS LANOLIN • *Water-free lanolin (wool fat).*

ANTI-OXIDANT • *A substance which prevents or slows the oxidising process of blended oils.*

ANTIBACTERIAL • *Any essential oil or mixture of essential oils capable of destroying harmful bacteria.*

BERGAMOT • *The essential oil distilled from the peel of the citrus fruit bergamot, a member of the orange tree family.*

CAJUPUT • *The essential oil extracted from the leaves and buds of the Malay kayu-puti, which grows abundantly throughout Malaysia and the Molucca Islands.*

CARRIER OIL/BASE OIL/VEGETABLE OIL • *Base oil to which has been added a quantity of pure essential oil.*

COLD-PRESSED • *A process by which the beneficial oil of a plant or seed is extracted without the use of heat.*

COMPRESS • *A piece of cloth soaked in a herbal infusion or a solution of water and essential oils.*

DENATURED • *To make alcohol unfit for drinking.*

ENFLEURAGE • *Extraction of the essential oil of a scented flower or herb by using salt and/or an odourless vegetable oil.*

ESSENTIAL OIL • *Volatile oil found in herbs and flowers, giving them their characteristic aroma and taste.*

FRIAR'S BALSAM • *See* Tincture of Benzoin.

MACERATION • *Extraction of essential oil of a flower by heating in an odourless vegetable oil.*

MODIFIER • *In perfume making modifiers are the top note essential oils which, when added to a perfume blend, give it an interesting 'twist'.*

NEROLI • *Bitter orange flower.*

NIAOULI • *The essence extracted by distillation from the bush* Melaleuca verdiflora. *It contains phenol, a powerful antibiotic and antiseptic.*

ORRISROOT • *Powder made from the root of some iris plants which absorbs and holds the fragrance of other herbs and flowers.*

ORRISROOT PERFUME BASE • *See* Orrisroot tincture.

ORRISROOT TINCTURE • *Solution of alcohol and orrisroot.*

SEBUM • *Secretion of the sebaceous glands.*

SIMMERING POT • *A small ceramic vessel with a candle inside. A small saucer containing a mixture of fragrant oil and water sits on top of the pot and the burning candle releases the oil's fragrant vapours.*

STEPHANOTIS • *Climbing tropical plant with fragrant white waxy flowers.*

TINCTURE OF BENZOIN • *Fragrant aromatic resin steeped in alcohol.*

TONIC • *Substance or mixture which has an overall beneficial or invigorating effect on the body system.*

VOLATILE ESSENCE • *Essence obtained from herbs and flowers by the process of distillation.*

VOLATILE OIL • *See* Essential oil.

# About the author

Alan Hayes' interest in herbs first began as a teenager, when he became aware, through his grandmother, of the herbal lore that had been passed down through the Hayes family for generations. Alan's interest grew as he studied herbal medicines and natural therapies, and his expertise expanded. On this basis, he has now established a reasonably self-sufficient lifestyle for himself and his family.

Using the knowledge gained from his study and from family records, Alan has become the successful author of a number of books on herbal lore and healing, notably the bestseller *It's So Natural*, an A to Z compilation of environmentally-friendly hints, tips and remedies for the home, health and garden, based on the author's widely syndicated and popular weekly column of the same name. More recently, Alan has published *Country Scents* and *Bath Scents* which bring the magic and colour of herbs into the home and garden, in easy-to-read, step-by-step formats that allow the reader to capture the charms of yesteryear with natural products.

With an ever growing number of people interested in natural health care, Alan has continued to write on this subject, so that others may benefit from his knowledge and experience in this fascinating area.